Sexual MINDFULNESS

DR. RICHARD BLONNA

APOCRYPHILE
PRESS

Apocryphile Press
1700 Shattuck Ave #81
Berkeley, CA 94709
www.apocryphilepress.com

Printed in the United States of America
ISBN 978-1-949643-08-4 | paperback
ISBN 978-1-949643-09-1 | epub

Table of Contents

Part 3: Sexual Mindfulness

This book is dedicated to Frank LaBruno

Part 1
Let’s Talk About Sex

Introduction

When I was a young man in my 20s I was always on the go and could never sit still very long. I had big plans and lots of energy to accomplish them. I remember always feeling that there was so much to do and so little time to do it. I think I spent about half of my time *thinking about* what I needed to do and most of the other half actually *doing* it. I don't think I spent more than 10 percent of my time actually *being* in the present moment. My thoughts were always drifting off into the past ("Why did this or that have to happen?" or "I wish I had done this or that differently") or the future ("I think I'll try this tomorrow" or "I better get ready for that next month").

I got a lot accomplished, advanced in my education and my career, and made some money. Throughout this period I never seemed to be very happy or aware of the present moment, content to just *be* myself. I was always in the process of *becoming* someone, never *being* myself.

At the time, my wife and I had a third-floor attic apartment that a *paisano* from my family was renting to us for a minimal amount. Frank and his wife Fanny were an old Italian couple from the same village in Italy as my father. Their grown children were married and had moved out and into houses of their own. Frank and Fanny were both well into their 80s at the time but had a vibrant quality that made them seem years younger. I think they enjoyed having Heidi and I on the third floor. It was like having their kids home again.

Frank had an amazing capacity for just *being* in the present moment. Although his three-story apartment building was in a very developed urban area, he had this amazing garden that took up most of his 800-square-foot yard. In his garden he planted tomatoes, peaches, figs, and other fruits, but his pride and joy were his grapes, from which he made wine in his basement. On more than a couple of occasions I enjoyed the pleasure of a lunch comprised of Fanny's homemade pasta with marinara sauce made from their tomatoes and Frank's wine that seemed to have the maximum alcohol achievable under normal fermentation.

I used to watch Frank walk in his garden: back and forth, back and forth, hands clasped behind his back, half-lit stogie in his mouth, pacing the same twenty-five-foot horizontal east-to-west path, pausing only to change directions and pace north to south. I remember saying to myself, "What a crazy old dude, all he ever does is pace *mindlessly* back and forth through his garden."

How silly I was. What I didn't realize then was that Frank's pacing was *anything but* mindless. I remember now how he would stop and lean his head back, eyes closed, nostrils flared, experiencing his garden through its aromas, moisture, and sounds. I recall how a thin smile would cross his face as he stopped to examine a grape, taste a fig, caress a tomato. His actions were hardly mindless.

What I now realize is that Frank epitomized mindfulness. *Everything* he did was mindful. It would frustrate me to watch him pick a tomato. He would carefully examine each fruit before he picked it, choosing only the ripest for Fanny's sauce. He would gently pluck the fruit from the vine, being oh so careful not to disturb the other pieces that were still ripening. Then he would hold the tomato up to the sunlight, wipe it off on his shirt, and examine it one last time before gently placing it in his basket. He would then move on to the next tomato, repeating the procedure. It could take him a good twenty minutes to pick the day's tomatoes. I would say to myself, "What a waste of time. I could have done that in five minutes." I think Frank realized how I felt because he would give me a knowing look, as if to say, "Slow down, Rich, and enjoy the full experience of these wonderful tomatoes, a gift to us from nature."

I miss those early evenings spent with Frank in his garden. How I wish he and Fanny were still around, so I could tell them how much I can now appreciate their simple, honest lives, and the mindfulness they brought to each moment. How much I would now give for a wordless walk in the garden with Frank, stopping now and then to smell the air, sift through the soil, and sit on the garden swing, merely *being* in the presence of such beauty.

Chapter 1

Let's Talk About Sex and Your Sexual Identity

Before we jump into discussing sexual mindfulness we need to answer the question, "What is sex?" You're probably wondering why I even need to ask the question because everyone knows what sex is, right? Well, maybe. Sex can mean many different things to different people. Still not convinced? Let me just share a little story that dates all the way back to 1998.

On January 16, 1998 President Bill Clinton infamously told the nation, "I did not have sexual relations with that woman, Miss Lewinsky," while at the same time admitting that the stains on her blue dress were there because she had performed oral sex on him in his office. At the time I was 47 years old and my first reaction to his quote was, "yeah, sure, so how do you explain the stains on her dress?" After thinking it over for a while I began to wonder if he really didn't think that oral sex was *sex*.

At the time I was teaching a Human Sexuality college course so I decided to ask my students. I was amazed at the results. Most *did not* consider oral sex, *sex*. They viewed it more as a type of foreplay or making out rather than putting it in the same class as intercourse. Furthermore, most of them who had given or received oral sex but hadn't had sexual intercourse considered themselves to be virgins.

To be honest, I was blown away by the results. I was only a few years younger than President Clinton at the time he made his statement and I definitely viewed oral sex as sex. In fact I viewed oral sex as not only a type of sex, but probably the *most intimate* form of sex because of the face to genital exposure someone has when performing it. In fact, I still feel this way.

So What is Sex?

Sex is a word derived from sexuality, a broader term that refers to all of the dimensions of being a sexual creature. Your sexuality is influenced by several factors. Some of the most powerful influences are biological, social, cultural, religious, moral, ethical, political, legal, economic, and psychological factors. You can take *any* aspect of your sexuality and explain it in terms of the influence of these factors.

Let's use birth control as an example. All you have to do is start with the term birth control itself . Most people use the terms birth control, contraception, and family planning interchangeably and assume they mean the same thing. Although the three terms are similar because they refer to strategies for preventing unintended pregnancy, they are vastly different in terms of their nature, scope, and acceptability to their advocates and foes.

Birth control is a broad term encompassing all methods designed to prevent pregnancy and birth. It includes all contraceptive methods, post-conceptive methods, and abortion, which is designed to interrupt an established pregnancy. Various religious and political groups who support preventing unintended pregnancies do not support birth control because it includes abortion.

Contraception refers to all methods designed to prevent conception or fertilization. Contraceptive methods work by preventing the sperm and egg from uniting to cause fertilization. While some groups might support contraception in general, they might be against public agencies or schools giving away free condoms because they believe that such behavior promotes acceptance of pre-marital sex (a term not supported by other groups).

Family planning implies the desire to have children at some point in time. Planning a family involves postponing childbearing until it is desired, spacing subsequent births and avoiding pregnancy at other times. Family planning does not refer to specific methods or techniques to avoid unintended pregnancy. It also doesn't take into account people who choose to have sex but never plan on having a family, getting married or committing to one partner. Such people might be opposed to the use of the term family planning because they feel it stigmatizes them.

Assuming that you could get over the naming barrier and get agreement from folks regarding their support of the goal of preventing unintended pregnancies, there would still be vast divides regarding *how* this goal is accomplished.

Economic factors influence everything— from what methods are developed (based on how profitable they are) and available on the market—to what you can afford to use consistently and correctly. While theoretically there is an affordable method for every sexually-active person, *social, cultural* and *psychological* factors influence whether or not people will purchase and use them. Public support (and tax dollars or other subsidies) for providing affordable methods to those who can't pay for them is divided.

Religious and Cultural factors are among the strongest influences on the use or non-use of methods designed to prevent unintended pregnancies. Cultural traditions and religious beliefs influence *moral* and *ethical* positions regarding sex and how to prevent unintended pregnancies. The religious, cultural, moral, and ethical beliefs of those in positions of power in government and industry influence the policies they promote regarding preventing unintended pregnancy.

Political and *legal* factors also come into play in the form of government testing and regulation. In the USA, the Food and Drug Administration (FDA) has rules and protocols for testing newly proposed birth control methods. Laws and legal debates such as the Roe vs Wade abortion decision impact the availability of methods and how they are made available to consumers like yourself.

You can take any aspect of human sexuality and explore it through the lens of these broad societal factors. That isn't the purpose of this book.

This book will focus on your personal sexuality and your sexual relationship, while understanding that these have not evolved in a vacuum. A big part of sexual mindfulness is understanding these influences without letting them control you or serve as barriers to having the kind of sex life you want and deserve. In this book we will focus on the one aspect of your sexuality that exerts the greatest influence on this—your *sexual identity.*

Your Sexual Identity

Your sexual identity is the comprehensive term used to describe how you see yourself and behave as a sexual person. Your sexual identity has six parts; (1) your biological sex/gender, (2) your gender identity, (3) your gender role, (4), your sexual orientation, (5) your sexual behavior, and (6) your sexual response. All six of these parts combine to form a picture of how you see yourself and behave as a sexual person (Blonna and Carter, 2018).

One way to view these parts is to look at them as five different continuums. To a certain extent these continuums are fluid and change over the course of your life. Some are more fluid than others.

Biological Continuum

Male	Intersex	Female

Gender Continuum (Gender Identity and Gender Role)

Masculine	Transgender	Feminine

Sexual Orientation Continuum

Heterosexual	Bisexual	Homosexual

Sexual Behavior Continuum

Not Interested	Average Interest	Very Interested

Sexual Response Continuum

Not Responsive	Average Response	Very Responsive

For example, your biological continuum is determined by your chromosomes (XX or XY) and your genetic inheritance. Your chromosomes and genetic inheritance determine things such as your biological sex/gender (male, female, intersex, other), internal and external sex organs, hormone type and levels, and your physical characteristics (body size, shape, hair and eye color, skin pigmentation, etc). These biological factors are fixed at conception and can only be changed through medical, surgical, or cosmetic interventions (Blonna, 2012).

I don't want to politicize this or make any moral judgments about it. What you make of these biologically-determined outcomes and how they influence the path you choose in life is your business. There is no denying, however, that biological events that will shape the course of your life start when sperm meets egg.

Unlike your biological continuum, the other continuums are more fluid.

Your gender continuum is very fluid and changes over the course of your life. How you see yourself (and act) as a man, woman, both, or neither changes as you age, grow, mature, and gain sexual and relationship experience. For many people the same holds true for their sexual orientation continuum. While the overwhelming percentage of people retain their initial sexual orientation throughout their lives, it is no longer unusual to hear of men or women in their adulthood, mid-life, or older adulthood becoming attracted to member of the same, opposite, or both sexes. In some cases they repressed these desires for decades and tried to conform to society's norms. In others, the spark of desire was more spontaneous.

Your sexual behavior continuum is very fluid. Your level of sexual desire will wax and wane over the course of your lifetime. Your sexual behavior repertoire will grow and change as you mature, enter into sexual relationships, and face or no longer face challenges associated with pregnancy and STD prevention issues.

Lastly, your sexual response continuum is also very fluid. Sexual response is the result of a complex interplay between your body, mind, and spirit. Becoming aroused and achieving orgasm are intimately related to your thoughts, feelings, physical health, mental well-being, and a host of other variables. These variables and others vary for each sexual encounter and change over time as a result of the aging process.

For example, I am a 67-year-old, white heterosexual man who has been married for 47 years and still enjoys sex with his wife. I understand the biological aspects of being male and how they are related to my sexual response. I know a lot about the internal and external parts of my sexual anatomy and how they work. I am aware of the effects of aging on things such as hormones, muscle mass, sexual response, etc., all components of being a biological male. I also am aware of how I see myself as a 67-year-old man. I understand and am happy with my gender role and how it has evolved over the years. I am comfortable being heterosexual and married and have a repertoire of satisfying sexual activities that I engage in by myself and with my wife. Lastly, I understand and am comfortable with my sexual response. I see how it has changed over the decades and do not see this change as something negative. It is just *different* and no less satisfying than it was when I was in my 20s.

I continue to practice formal and informal mindfulness activities on a regular basis and they help me stay aware of all aspects of my sexuality and the rest of my life. I try to make the most of the present moment because I am aware that it is the only moment that I have. The past is gone and the future is yet to happen.

Sexual mindfulness will help you do the same. It will help you become more aware of your sexual identity and understand how the different parts interact and contribute to your sexual satisfaction or dissatisfaction. In order to better understand *your* sexual identity and sexual mindfulness you need to know how your mind thinks about sex.

You need to understand both the *process* of how your mind thinks about sex as well as the *content* of that thinking. In the next chapter we'll take a slight detour away from our discussion of your sexual identity to explore how your mind thinks about sex in general. We'll then return to exploring your sexual identity armed with a better understanding of the role your mind plays in it.

Chapter 2

How Your Mind Thinks About Sex

One of the hardest things for me to understand when I started practicing mindfulness was the role played by my mind. I really didn't even understand the difference between the brain and the mind. During my first formal training program in Acceptance and Commitment Therapy (ACT), I was continually corrected by the instructor when I made statements about the brain that actually were related to the mind. A big part of ACT training is learning how to separate yourself from what your mind is telling you about a particular situation. This allows you to step back and assess what your mind is telling you more objectively.

The best analogy I can think of to explain the relationship between your brain and your mind is the relationship between your computer and the software it runs. Your brain is similar to the computer. It is the structure that houses the software and makes it run. Your mind is like your computer's software. Just as your computer houses several different programs, so does your mind. While your computer might have a word processing program, a photo and video viewing program, an internet gateway program and several others, your mind has its own programs.

Your mind's "programs" are your thoughts, feelings, self-talk (also known as personal scripts), and mental images (Hayes, 2005, Hayes et al, 1999, 2001). While you're familiar with thoughts and feelings, let me take a moment to define what personal scripts and mental images are.

Your personal scripts (also known as your self-talk) about sex can be compared to scenes in a movie. The movie in this case is your sex life, and each personal script paints a picture of how your mind recalls the scene playing out. What you tell yourself about these scenes is your sexual self-talk. You have personal scripts about every aspect of your sexuality going all the way back to your earliest recollections and use of language. Your mind is capable of bringing these scripts into the present moment and projecting them forward when confronted with a new sexual situation.

Mental images are the pictures you see when you close your eyes and think about your sexual personal scripts. If the scripts are the dialogue in your movie, the mental images are the pictures that go along with it. Your mental images, like your personal scripts and thoughts and emotions, are based on past experiences and your earliest recollections of being a sexual person.

The other key similarity between your brain/mind and your computer/software is the ability of your mind and your computer to run several programs simultaneously. At any given time your computer is running its operating system, virus checker, email, etc. Your mind does the same thing. It simultaneously thinks, feels, and responds to external stimuli such as sights, sounds, smells etc. when you are in a sexual situation. Not only can your computer and your brain run these programs simultaneously, they are capable of running them non-stop 24/7 every day. In other words, your mind is a non-stop 24/7 thinking and feeling machine. And people wonder why we think about sex so much???

Lastly, just as your computer's programs can get corrupted, work erratically and cause your whole computer to freeze, your mind's programs can get corrupted, function erratically, and cause your mind to freeze and not think properly.

An ACT-Based Approach

Most of what I have learned about the mind was through my post-doctoral training in Acceptance and Commitment Therapy (ACT), Morita Therapy, and Naikan Self-Reflection. ACT is considered the third wave of Cognitive Behavior Therapy (CBT), which focuses on the role your thoughts and feelings play in driving your behavior (Hayes, 2005). Morita and Naikan are two forms of Japanese psychology that have strong grounding in Buddhism. A common thread in these three forms of therapy is mindfulness (Krech, 2002).

Steven Hayes is the creator of ACT. Hayes and his colleagues (Hayes, et al, 1999, 2001) at the University of Nevada at Reno found that when you learn something, you learn it *in relation to* other things specific to that time and place. In other words, all of your learning takes place within a certain *context;* it is contextual in nature. The context includes external factors (the time, place, and environment), as well as personal factors (age, experience etc.). ACT stresses the importance of the *context* of your learning, as well as the *content* of it.

For example, your current thoughts, feelings, self-talk, mental images, and behavior about a sexual situation are linked to its original context. ACT calls this context the original frame of reference or *relational frame.* A relational frame is the context from your past in which you were first exposed to (learned) the sexual experience. The way you respond to a current sexual situation is influenced by your mind's ability to use information from that original frame of reference, bring it into the present moment, and then project it forward and think about all of the possible ways it can play out. I call this *"going past, present, future."* Your mind's ability to go past, present, future, can either be helpful or unhelpful as you try to navigate a current sexual situation.

Let's use the first time you had sexual intercourse as an example. Your first episode of sexual intercourse occurred in a certain context. It took place at a certain time, with a specific person, in a designated place, and was linked to specific thoughts, feelings, personal scripts, and mental images. You were a certain age, at a specific point in your development, and had a certain level of sexual and relationship experience. All of these factors combined to form the context of that first sexual intercourse experience and this context is forever embedded in your mind.

This initial relational frame may have been a positive learning experience that evokes fond memories, emotions, and mental images—or it might have been a negative one that brings up troubling thoughts and self-talk, and painful emotions and mental images that you'd rather forget. If it was positive, it will more than likely help you navigate your current sexual situation. If the context was negative, filled with troubling thoughts and painful feelings and images, it can create a barrier to navigating a new sexual situation.

To illustrate this, let's look at Sharon, one of my former clients, and her earliest recollection of the first time she had sexual intercourse. Sharon was 36 years old when I spoke to her about this. She told me that she was a 15-year-old freshman in high school when she had sexual intercourse for the first time. Her partner, James, was 18, and a senior in the same school. James played on the football team and Sharon was a JV cheerleader when they met. Sharon recalls that she matured early and looked more like an 18-year-old senior than a 15-year-old freshman. James and Sharon were smitten with each other the first time they met. They started dating towards the end of her freshman year and things progressed from making out to heavy petting and oral sex pretty rapidly. Although Sharon had never had sexual intercourse before, she had given and received oral sex a few times in middle school and was eager to "do the deed," to use her words. By the July 4th weekend that summer they had sexual intercourse for the first time.

Sharon was an only child and her mother and father both worked fulltime until 6:00pm. James had a nearby part-time job that ended at 3:00pm. Sharon remembers that she was the one who initiated sexual intercourse. She really wanted to do it and told James to come over after work because she had a special treat for him. When he showed up at her door she had a skimpy halter top and tight shorts on that left very little to the imagination.

When James arrived and saw Sharon's outfit and the look on her face he became instantly aroused and before he could even put his stuff down Sharon started kissing him and grinding her pubic area against his. After a few minutes of this she literally dragged him into her bedroom and onto her bed where they continued to make out and grind against each other. She proceeded to take off her clothes and then started in on James. By the time she got James' shirt and pants off and started pulling down his underwear she noticed that he had lost his erection and had a very sheepish look on his face. She didn't realize what had happened until she looked at his underwear and realized he had prematurely ejaculated before even getting his clothes off.

She recalls feeling "really weird," like she had done something wrong and caused James to feel embarrassed. She remembers that he wanted to leave but she told him it was ok, maybe if they just made out a little he would get another erection and she could finally lose her virginity. James relented and they slowed things down a bit. Sharon recalled, "It is funny, but talking to you about this I can actually remember the whole thing vividly. I remember how James smelled, kind of a sour smell. I guess it was a combination of his sweat, semen, and not having showered after work. It was kind of gross. I also remember there was a song playing on the radio in the background that James just loved and I really hated. I even remember the feeling of his beard stubble on my face."

Sharon continued, "Well, anyway, James didn't take too long to get another erection but it turned out that he really didn't know what to do with it. He had a real hard time putting a condom on and it took him a long time to find my vaginal opening and put his penis in it. By that time I had lost some of my lubrication and the whole experience wasn't really that much fun. It actually hurt a little but I was determined to lose my virginity so we kept going. Actually, we didn't keep going for too long, because once again James came too soon."

"After the second time he just got frustrated and wanted to go home. I have to admit that I was kind of glad to see him leave. I couldn't wait to jump in the shower and wash his scent off of me and then call my best friend Maria and tell her all about it. All in all I was happy to lose my virginity, but the experience was not that great. It kind of made me not want to have intercourse for a while. James stopped calling me the next week and we eventually split up before the summer's end. He wound up going away to college and never returned to our town."

Sharon's experience with James was her initial frame of reference for sexual intercourse. The memory is tucked away in the recesses of her brain and can be recalled at a moment's notice. Another important thing to understand about this is that when Sharon recalls this learning frame or describes it as she did to me, she's referring to her *mind's version* of the experience. This is a *version* of the event, not the actual event. The ACT literature emphasizes that you can get into trouble when you believe that your *thoughts* about something are the same thing as your *actual experience* of the event. Any time you think about the past it is always subject to forgetfulness or embellishment. In other words, much of the detail is forgotten and what you do remember you tend to blow out of proportion—especially if it makes you look good.

Your past frames of reference always operate in the background of your brain just waiting to come to the surface when a new or similar sexual experience presents itself. This happens because your mind wants to protect you from harm. It wants you to really think about what happened the last time before taking action in the present moment. Understanding this and accepting it are key components of working *with* your mind instead of *against* it.

All Thoughts Are Not Created Equal

Another big part of my ACT training was learning to not take all of my thoughts so seriously. As a college professor, this was really hard to accept at first. For over 40 years of my life I had prized my intelligence and thinking abilities. Now I was being told to not take my thoughts so seriously. I wondered, "What is going on here???"

What I found out was that most of us tend to believe what our minds tell us about situations and we act on this information without questioning it too much. We tend to lump all of our thoughts together as being equally important and therefore pay *equal attention* to everything. This can really get us into trouble when thinking about sex.

In fact, all of our thoughts are *not* equal. For the purpose of narrowing this down, there are three kinds of thoughts: (1) helpful, (2) unhelpful or (3) benign. In terms of sex, helpful thoughts assist you in meeting your sexual and relationship goals. Unhelpful thoughts create barriers to doing this. Benign thoughts do not affect your goals one way or the other. A lot of benign thoughts are downright silly. If you track your thoughts for a few weeks you'll see that the majority of your self-talk falls into the latter two categories, especially when it concerns sex. For some crazy reason, most of us are not too logical when it comes to thinking about sex.

Mindfulness training helps you look at the *helpfulness* and *usefulness* of your thoughts in relation to your values and goals. ACT refers to this as *values-congruent behavior*. In other words, your sexual actions are consistent with your values. You'll see later on in the book why it is important to understand your sexual values and always consider them when setting sexual or relationship goals (Hayes, 2005). To help determine what's useful and what isn't, consider this basic question: *"Are these thoughts helping me act in ways that are consistent with my values and goals?"* If your answer is yes, you can accept them and continue to move forward. If the answer is no, it is perfectly OK to acknowledge this and dismiss those thoughts as unhelpful because they don't help you behave in ways that are consistent with your values and goals. You can literally stop and say to yourself: "*That is not a very helpful thought. I'm not going to let it guide how I react.*"

What can you do to break free from unhelpful thoughts, feelings, and self-talk? One way is to start viewing your mind as a computer. This simple exercise, *Your Mind as a Computer,* will help you do this.

Mind Exercise # 1: Your Mind as a Computer

As a 24/7 thinking and feeling machine, your mind is constantly going past, present, and future when you are confronted by a new sexual situation. The following exercise is designed to help you accept the unhelpful ways your mind thinks about new situations and shift your focus off of this and onto productive behavior.

Instructions:

1. Describe a new sexual situation that has gotten you stuck and is triggering troubling thoughts or painful emotions.
2. Tell yourself the following three things:

   "Like my phone apps and computer programs, a lot of the information from the programs my mind runs are not helpful or very accurate, and can actually create barriers that contribute to me getting stuck in a sexual rut .

   "It is OK for me ignore these unhelpful thoughts and feelings when they stand in the way of meeting my sexual goals."

   "It is not very productive to try to figure out 'why' my mind is creating these barriers. It is more efficient to shift my focus off of these unhelpful mental programs and onto doing something that moves me forward towards my values-based sexual goals."

In time you will stop wasting so much time trying to figure out *why* your mind behaves the way it does and focus on *what* it is telling you and *whether* this information is *helpful* or not. You'll learn to laugh at your mind rather than take it so seriously and allow it to trigger a stress response.

Common Thinking Traps

In *The Happiness Trap*, Russ Harris (2007), a famous ACT-based therapist, physician, and writer describes common thinking traps that most people fall into. These thinking traps contribute to psychological distress and can create barriers that cause you to get stuck in a sexual rut. Getting stuck in these thinking traps makes it very hard to be mindful and focused on the present moment. In this section I'll briefly discuss a few of my favorite thinking traps and how to become more mindful of them, see them coming, and manage them.

The "Thoughts Are Reality" Trap

The "thoughts are reality" trap is based on the notion that your thoughts about a sexual situation represent the objective reality of the situation. In fact, your thoughts about the sexual situation are just that, your *thought about it.* The only way to know the reality of a sexual situation is to experience it directly, firsthand. You fall into the trap when you think your thoughts about a sexual situation or event are the same thing as the actual situation or event.

Let's use group sex as an example. Imagine that you've been online viewing some short XXX-rated video clips of group sex. You find yourself getting excited and you say to yourself; "*Wow that is hot. I'd really enjoy doing it. Maybe I can get my girlfriend to go along with this.*" In fact, most people cannot handle being involved in group sex by themselves, let alone with their partner participating. When they actually directly experience the situation they find out that the reality of it is very different from what their mind has told them about it.

The Old, Outdated Thoughts and Scripts Trap

As I discussed previously, everyone carries around outdated thoughts and personal scripts about themselves. Many of these are related to sex and are accompanied by outdated mental images. Like photographs of how you looked twenty years ago, they've contributed to who you are, but they're often just faded representations of your past. In many cases, these faded snapshots and the thoughts that accompany them are no longer based on the reality of who you are as a person in the present moment. Lying just below the surface like land mines ready to explode when you step on them, these outdated thoughts and personal scripts can sabotage your best efforts to deal with new sexual situations.

Take the case of Sharon. The reason she came to see me was that her outdated thoughts and personal scripts about a failed relationship were keeping her from moving forward in a new one with a guy she met and really liked. Whenever she was with him all she could think of and see was her ex-fiancée asking for her engagement ring because he was ending the relationship. It took time for her to accept that the reasons for the break-up had more to do with his issues than with her. In fact, in the six years since the break-up she had grown as a person. The experience of that failed relationship had made her much stronger and clearer about what she wanted in a new one. She came to realize that her old, outdated sexual scripts related to her failed relationship no longer represented the person she is now.

The "I Can Figure It All Out in My Head" Trap

The "I Can Figure It All Out in My Head" Trap is based on the notion that you do not need to experience something directly to figure it out in advance. It is a trap because, as we discussed previously, your thoughts about something are just that, your thoughts. They may or may not match up to the reality of something after you have experienced it first-hand. Many people fall into this trap because they want to avoid potentially painful experiences. They are afraid to get hurt again so they ruminate endlessly about how a certain situation will play out.

Unfortunately, this plays right into worsening the problem, because your mind would like nothing better than to protect you from harm by having you sit back and let it run away endlessly. Remember, your mind is a 24/7 thinking and feeling machine. For every "solution" it comes up with, it creates ten new "what if?" questions.

Take Sharon's case again. She can sit back and try to figure everything out about her new romantic attraction and refuse to go on another date until she "figures out everything" that could go right or wrong. Unfortunately, she is deluding herself because whatever her mind tells her is only words until they actually spend time together and she has the chance to experience how the relationship plays out. You fall into the "I Can Figure It All Out in My Head Trap" when you think that you can avoid direct experience and rely on what your mind tells you about a new situation.

We all fall into these thinking traps every once in a while. Most of us tend to fall into some traps more than others without even realizing it. One way to be more mindful of these traps is to start paying more attention to them. Realizing that you are falling into a thinking trap takes practice. The following exercise, *My Thinking Trap Journal*, will help you to keep track of the thinking and feeling traps associated with your sexual thinking

Mind Exercise # 2: My Thinking Trap Journal

Instructions:

1. Begin keeping this journal tomorrow.
2. Keep the journal at least five days a week for a few weeks.
3. Rotate the five days so both weekdays and weekends are accounted for.
4. Keep this in whatever format you desire—electronic, lined paper, bound journal etc.
5. Fill it in whenever it is convenient for you; as they occur, at the end of the day, first thing in the morning, etc.

6. Don't let more than a day pass when recording a thinking trap. This will keep the details of it from blurring. Focus on the three traps discussed in this chapter.
7. Use the following Format:

Date:
Event that Triggered the Trap: What was the event that triggered your thinking?
Thinking trap: Cite the specific trap you fell into as labeled in the chapter.
What did your mind tell you about it?: Write down your actual self-talk about the event.
What feelings did your mind trigger?: Describe the emotions that your mind triggered.
How did your body react?: Describe the physical effects of the trap on your body.
How Did You Behave after You Fell Into the Trap?: Describe the actions you took after falling into the trap.

Example:
Event That Triggered the Trap: "I was asked to go on a blind date with friends."
Thinking trap: "I fell into the I Can Figure It Out... Trap."
What did your mind tell you about it?: "I'm going to write down lists of all of the good and bad things that could possibly happen if I go out on this date and then decide if I am going to accept."
What feelings did your mind trigger?: "I got very anxious."
How did your body react?: "I felt nauseous and had tension in my neck."
How Did You Behave after You Fell Into the Trap?: "I took a Xanax to calm down."

In time, you will understand which traps you are most likely to fall into, the circumstances that trigger them, and how your body, mind, and behavior are affected by them. You can use this knowledge to become mindful of the situations that trigger your sexual thinking traps as well as the outdated thoughts and personal scripts associated with them. This can help you avoid some of them and prepare for the rest. You can also use it to create more healthy coping strategies to deal with the situations that trigger the traps. For the example cited, instead of popping a Xanax, maybe you could go for a run or mow the lawn.

In time, you will be able to recognize when you are about to fall into a thinking trap and actually prevent it from happening. Learning to accept how your mind works and the traps it occasionally falls into takes training.

Chapter 3

Your Biological Sex/Gender

In this book we'll use the terms biological sex and biological gender interchangeably. They both refer to the biological aspects of sexual identity. Your biological sex focuses on your genetic inheritance and your sexual anatomy (actual body parts) and physiology (sexual chemistry). You have thoughts, feelings, self-talk, and mental images linked to all aspects of your biological gender. They can be helpful or unhelpful in accepting who you are as a sexual person.

Just think about the inner dialogue you have at times related to *anatomical* issues such as the size and shape of your body and specific parts (penis, breasts, hips etc.), the color and texture of your hair, the color and size of your eyes, the whiteness of your teeth, and the nature of your smile.

How about *physiological* issues? What have you told yourself about your hormones, hot flashes, menstrual cycle, sexual desire, or the nature and frequency of your erections (or lack of them)? The sheer number of troubling thoughts, painful emotions, negative self-talk and mental images that most people have related to their sexual anatomy and physiology is staggering. If you multiply the number of unhelpful thoughts and feelings about these issues by the number of adults in first-world countries where people have some disposable income, you can begin to estimate the market for products and services designed to help people eliminate concerns about their sexual anatomy and physiology. Stress over sexual anatomy and physiology issues has fueled the fashion, cosmetics, weight loss, and cosmetic surgery industries, just to name a few.

Around the world, men and women spend billions of dollars each year trying to "improve" parts of their bodies that work perfectly well but are the source of troubling thoughts, painful emotions, and negative self-talk and mental images. Millions of people just like you have been brainwashed into believing that they do not look, smell, or function well enough to have a satisfying sex life.

The cosmetic surgery industry has tried to convince you that you could attract partners or enjoy sex more if only you had new breasts, a new nose, chin, waist, etc. etc. The weight loss industry tries to convince you that you are too fat and that if you had washboard abdominal muscles you would have a more satisfying sex life and a healthier sexual identity. The sexual enhancement industry tries to make you (and your partners) believe that if you could muster "3-hour erections" (an actual side-effect warning issued during a commercial for a commonly used treatment for erectile disorder) this will solve all of your sexual and relationship problems. The fashion industry tries to convince you that if you wear certain clothes or have specific "accessories" (jewelry, watches, belts, bags, etc.) it will create a powerful sexual aura that will have sexy men and women falling over themselves trying to get to you first. If you are a woman, the lingerie industry wants you to believe that wearing a bra that costs $150 will somehow transform your breasts into the ticket to a fulfilling sex life.

These are just some examples of the thoughts, feelings, self-talk, and mental images that you might have that are related to your sexual anatomy and physiology. What are your thoughts and feelings related to these issues? Are they helpful and consistent with your sexual values and relationship goals? Are they unhelpful and contribute to your being stuck in a sexual rut?

In the rest of this book I'll teach you how to become more mindful of such sexual thoughts and feelings and how to coexist with them without getting stuck. The following two exercises are designed to help you be more mindful of your sexual anatomy and physiology and how they contribute to your sexual happiness.

Biological Sex Exercise # 1: Body Image Inventory (Male and Female)

Purpose: Body image refers to your evaluation and perception of your body, specific body parts, and their functioning. It includes the messages (positive and negative) that you tell yourself about your body and your sexual self-esteem. The following inventory will help you assess your body image.

Instructions:

Rate each body part listed below using the following scale: extremely satisfied = 5; satisfied = 4; neutral = 3; dissatisfied = 2; extremely dissatisfied = 1.

1. eyes ________
2. nose ________
3. hair ________
4. ears ________
5. teeth ________
6. mouth ________
7. weight ________
8. shoulders ________
9. chest /breasts ________
10. arms ________
11. calves ________
12. hands ________
13. height ________
14. stomach ________
15. buttocks ________
16. hips ________
17. thighs ________
18. feet ________
19. sex organs ________
20. overall body ________

Scoring:

105–80 Very positive body image
60–80 Positive body image
40–60 Ambivalent about your body
20–40 Negative body image
0–20 Very negative body image

Answer the following questions:

1. What are your thoughts, self-talk, mental images and feelings about your body?
2. How do these mind programs contribute to your sexual problems and/or keep you stuck in your sexual rut?

Hang on to this body image inventory and the answers to the questions. In the second half of the book you'll learn how to use sexual mindfulness techniques to co-exist with your troubling thoughts and painful emotions as you move forward towards meeting your sexual and relationship goals. The next exercise looks at societal messages related to body image and how they impact your sexual identity.

Biological Sex Exercise # 2: Society and Body Image

Purpose: Body image is a key component of gender identity and gender role. This activity explores societal messages about body image. These messages, whether overt or covert, are often at odds with your sexual values and contribute to getting stuck.

Instructions:

1. Describe three specific overt messages you have received regarding what your body "should" look like. Cite three different sources (husband, wife, partner, parents, friends, etc.)

2. Give three examples of covert (TV, magazines, etc.) body image messages that you've received from society.
3. Give three specific examples of adornment (clothing, accessories, etc.) and grooming (make-up, hair, etc.) that you've received regarding how you should look.
4. What are your thoughts, self-talk, mental images and feelings about this?
5. How do these societal expectations impact your current satisfaction with your sexual identity?

CHAPTER 4

Your Gender Identity and Gender Role

Your gender identity and gender role are flip sides of the same coin. Your gender identity is how you see yourself as a man or a woman (or both or neither). It is your ***internal picture*** of what it means to be a man, woman, etc., and contains your thoughts, feelings, self-talk, and mental images related to your biological gender.

Your gender role is your ***outward portrayal*** of your gender identity and biological sex. It involves the way you dress, your hair style, make-up, your choice of friends, career, education, and many other issues that show the world how you portray your internal picture of what it means to be a man or woman (or both or neither). Your gender role is the action part of this dyad because it relates to how you *behave* in relation to your gender identity.

Your gender identity begins at birth as you are welcomed into the world by your parent(s). They will use words like son or daughter, boy or girl, and dress you in clothes that they feel are appropriate for your biological sex. Some people call this assigning gender. In actuality it is *assigning gender identity*. Remember—your biological gender is determined by your genetic inheritance and chromosomes, not what your parents tell you. There is a long history of research that shows that biological males and females are treated differently (played with, spoken to, dressed, etc.) based on their biological sex and subsequent gender assignment.

Your gender identity continues to develop by listening to and observing the men and women in your family and culture and being exposed to peers and the media. By age three you develop a sense of what it means to be a boy or girl or other. Much of your gender identity development is overt (people telling you what to say and how to act) and the rest is covert (being exposed to societal expectations through the media). For example, your mom and dad give you overt messages by telling you how you should look, think and behave in specific situations. Peer groups exert incredible pressure to conform to their norms. This is true for traditional young men and women as well as transgender youth (Blonna and Carter, 2018).

Advertising is a great example of how mass culture conveys covert messages about what it means to be a man or woman. Advertisements for clothing, cars, fragrances, beer, and a thousand other things show images of men and women oozing sexuality. These infer that if you only look like or act this way you can be just like the people in the advertisement.

These overt and covert messages are not necessarily bad if they are consistent with how you see yourself and mesh with your sexual values and goals. They can be a major source of sexual pain and suffering, however, when they come in conflict with how you see yourself and with your sexual values and relationship goals. This is why a big part of sexual mindfulness training focuses on understanding what your mind is telling you about your gender identity in the present moment.

These values conflicts often occur when you *compare yourself* to peer, societal, and cultural standards that don't mesh with your own. Most of my students and clients are stuck on sexual issues because they compare themselves to someone else's standards that they either cannot meet or do not want to meet. Sexual mindfulness training can teach you how to quiet your troubled mind when it engages in unhelpful comparisons of any nature, especially those related to sex. Comparing your sexuality against others' and judging the quality of your sex life based on what others say and do is a prescription for getting stuck. This book will show you how to let your own values and goals be the measure against which you judge your sexual thoughts, feelings, and behavior. In reality, the only judging that is helpful is when you judge whether or not your thoughts and feelings are helpful or unhelpful in staying true to your values, taking action, and meeting your sexual goals.

As previously mentioned, your gender role is your outward portrayal of your gender identity and biological sex. It involves the way you dress, your hair style, make-up, your choice of friends, career, education, and many other issues that show the world how you portray your internal picture of what it means to be a man or woman (or both or neither). Your gender role is the action part of your sexual identity. It is how you *behave* in relation to your gender identity, biological sex, and sexual orientation. There is no one correct gender role. The correct gender role is the one that meshes with what you value about being a man or woman (or both or neither) and how this factors into your relationships. Being a "traditional male" or "feminist woman" or any other type of gender role is neither good nor bad, it just *is*. The most important thing is whether or not it works for you and your sexual and relationship values and goals.

Unfortunately, many people adopt a gender role that is inconsistent with their personal values and goals because they try to please others or meet societal standards that do not reflect who they are. If you do this it will surely cause you to get stuck in relationships and sexual behaviors that are unsatisfying and do not mesh with your values and goals.

Gender Identity Exercise # 1: Messages About Gender

Purpose: The purpose of this activity is to help you become more mindful of the thoughts, feelings, self-talk, and mental images you've developed regarding your gender identity and gender role by examining the messages you received about these things throughout your life up to this point. This is the starting point for learning how to coexist with unhelpful sexual thoughts and feelings related to your gender identity and gender role.

Instructions

1. For each of the stages of life below describe one specific message you received regarding what was expected of you as a man/woman, boy/girl during that phase in your life. You might find it helpful to look through old family photo albums, school yearbooks and other sources to help you remember that phase of your life.

    - early childhood (0-5 years old)
    - childhood (6-10 years old)
    - early adolescence (11-14 years old)
    - adolescence (15-19 years old)
    - young adulthood (19-25 years old)
    - adulthood (25-45 years old)
    - middle adulthood (45-65 years old)
    - older adulthood (65 + years old)

2. After describing what was expected of you during this time, comment on what was expected of the opposite gender. Cite personal examples of what was expected of you compared to your opposite sex sibling if you had a brother or sister.
3. Describe the source of the message (parents, family, friends, etc.) and the context (where, when, and how it was delivered).
4. How did you behave in relation to these gender messages?
5. How has your gender identity and gender role changed over the years?
6. How do your thoughts, self-talk, mental images, and emotions influence your current gender role ?

This information can be used to complete other exercises later in the book. You can learn how to coexist with outdated sexual thoughts, feelings, self-talk and mental images that contribute to keeping you stuck in a sexual rut.

Chapter 5

Your Sexual Orientation/Preference

The two terms sexual orientation and sexual preference are often used synonymously. I prefer the term sexual orientation because I feel that it is broader and encompasses the term sexual preference. Your sexual orientation is your adult free choice of sexual partners.

I use the qualifier "adult," because it is not unusual for people to experiment with same and opposite sex partners in childhood, adolescence, and young adulthood. By adulthood people have had the time and opportunity to make an informed choice about the kinds of partners they desire and prefer to have sex with.

I use the qualifying term "free choice" because it eliminates sexual experiences that were forced, or occurred while incarcerated or in any other situation where free choice was curtailed.

There is no inherently right or wrong, or good or bad sexual orientation. No one knows why people have the sexual orientation they do. As with other preferences (food, career, political etc.) you are drawn to your sexual partners because they appeal to you and spark your sexual desire. No one knows for sure why this is so. There is no conclusive scientific evidence that links sexual orientation to hormones, parenting styles, dominant fathers, etc. It is not the purpose of this book to argue in favor of one type of sexual orientation over another. I am much more interested in helping you examine the thoughts, feelings, self-talk, and mental images you have of your sexual orientation and whether or not these are helpful or unhelpful in reaching sexual and relationship goals that are consistent with your values.

For example, imagine you are a gay or lesbian person and you value marriage and parenthood. Your sexual and relationship goals are to marry your partner and adopt two children. Even though this is becoming more common in America and other industrialized first-world countries, you still would not be in the mainstream and could face discrimination and other road blocks in achieving your goals. If you got stuck in trying to meet your goals, I would have you examine the helpfulness or unhelpfulness of your thoughts, feelings, self-talk, and mental images related to your goals. If these were unhelpful I would work with you in learning how to coexist with them while taking values-congruent action to get unstuck. In other words, I'd show you how you could continue to do what you needed to do to get married and adopt kids while bringing your unhelpful thoughts and feelings along for the ride rather than waste a lot of time and energy trying to change them.

Sexual Orientation Exercise # 1: My Sexual Orientation

Purpose: The purpose of this activity is to increase your awareness of your thoughts, personal scripts, mental images, and emotions related to your sexual orientation and how this contributes to being stuck in a sexual relationship rut.

Instructions:

1. Describe your sexual orientation in as much detail as you can.
2. Describe your thoughts, self-talk, mental images, and emotions about your sexual orientation.
3. Describe where your thoughts, feelings, etc. related to your sexual orientation are helpful and consistent with your biological gender, gender identity, and gender role.
4. Describe where these mind programs are unhelpful and contribute to being stuck in a sexual relationship rut.

CHAPTER 6

Your Sexual Behavior

While this is not a book about sexual technique, it is important to understand the full range of "sexual" behaviors because your mind has already developed thoughts, feelings, self-talk, and mental images about them that may be contributing to getting or staying stuck. Some of these thoughts, feelings, etc. about specific sexual behaviors may be outdated or based on common thinking traps that cause you to get stuck in a sexual rut.

For example, imagine you want to experiment with different forms of sexual fantasy with your current partner. Unfortunately your mind has created unhelpful scripts and mental images about sexual fantasy from past experiences and relationships. Some of these sexual fantasy scripts tell you things like, "it is perverted to fantasize about having group sex," or "you must really want to be abused if you fantasize about being tied up during sex," or "it is weird to dress up in different costumes during sex as part of a fantasy." Understanding the true nature of sexual fantasies and the pros and cons of acting them out in real life can help you create new thoughts, feelings, self-talk, etc. about them that will help you and your partner decide their place in your relationship.

A second reason for spending time discussing specific sexual activities is to help you appreciate the range of different sexually pleasurable things you can do by yourself or with a partner. Sometimes people, especially those in or contemplating monogamous relationships, worry about becoming bored. They fear that having just one partner will be unsatisfying because it is too sexually limiting. One of the main reasons for practicing sexual mindfulness is that it demonstrates how that kind of thinking is not only limiting and can contribute to you getting stuck sexually, it is also untrue. The range of sexually pleasurable activities available to you, regardless of your relationship status, is limited only by what your mind tells you about your limitations.

Your Sexual Continuum

One way to present the many forms of sexual behavior available to you is to place them on a continuum from the least intimate to the most intimate. This continuum starts with celibacy and ends with anal intercourse.

- Celibacy/abstinence
- Kissing/making out
- Petting/fondling
- Masturbation/fantasy (autoerotic behavior) A* and P**
- Sex toy use/fantasy (autoerotic behavior) A and P
- Cunnilingus
- Fellatio
- Analingus
- Vaginal intercourse
- Anal intercourse

* alone
** partnered (Blonna, 2012).
I will only touch on some of these behaviors in this chapter because I will go over them in detail in chapters 14-17.

Celibacy and Abstinence

Celibacy is defined as abstaining from sexual intercourse. If you are like most people you probably assume that celibacy and abstinence mean total avoidance of all forms of sexual release and the absence of sexual desire. In fact, celibacy may or may not include masturbation and fantasy as forms of sexual release. Celibate people also have varying degrees of sexual desire. Not all celibate people lack sexual interest and desire. Many have strong levels of desire but choose to channel their energy and desire into something other than sexual activities. They often do this out of a religious or spiritual commitment but can also choose to channel this energy into work, athletic activities, or other pursuits. People choose to be celibate for a variety of reasons.

Priests and nuns, for example, declare a vow of celibacy so they may devote themselves fully to serving God and never marry. It is a conscious, willful diversion of sexual energy into nonsexual activity. Celibate monks are able to transform sexual energy into a sense of deep caring and love that is unique and very powerful.

Many people do not choose to be celibate as part of a religious commitment. Some are simply not ready to begin having intercourse, and they choose to satisfy their sexual needs through other behaviors. Everyone develops sexually at a different pace. For example, you might have been ready for sexual intercourse at an earlier or later age than your friends. There is no absolute timeline for when it is the right time to become sexually active with other people.

You might also choose celibacy because you need time to recover or grieve from a bad relationship that ended painfully. You need time to heal emotionally and are not interested in having a sexual relationship with anybody. You might also choose celibacy because you do not have the time or the energy to get involved sexually with another person. You might feel that you need to devote all of your time and energy to school or work, especially if you are beginning a new career or just starting school.

Abstinence is similar to celibacy but does not mean the same thing. Abstinence refers to self-restraint or self-denial of some or all sexual activities. Abstinence does not necessarily mean denial of all forms of sexual behavior. For example, if you were in a situation and you did not have a condom you could choose to abstain from having unprotected intercourse but not some other form of sexual behavior, such as masturbation or oral sex. In addition, abstinence usually is not discussed as a lifelong spiritual or religious commitment.

Abstinence is more situational. You could choose to abstain for a day, a week, a month, a semester, and so on. You've probably already voluntarily chosen to abstain from sex at different times in your life. Maybe you were sick, or out of town on business, or away performing your military service. Once your mind starts to view abstinence as a situational choice and not a lifetime commitment, it can begin to form new, more helpful relational frames about it as a viable form of sexual expression, a choice to abstain from certain things at certain times.

Non-Penetrative Sexual Activities

Non-penetrative sexual activities offer a wide variety of pleasurable behaviors that can be carried out to the point of orgasm and involve little risk of pregnancy or disease. Non-penetrative sexual activity is often referred to as "outer-course" because it does not involve sexual penetration of the vagina, rectum, or mouth. Outer-course includes options ranging from kissing and hugging to using non-penetrative sex toys such as vibrators.

Kissing

As you have probably already found out, kissing can provide intense sensual and sexual delight. The sucking, licking, rubbing, and tongue probing associated with kissing someone can be very pleasurable and carries no risk of pregnancy. As many people age, however, they become more genitally focused and lose some of their interest in kissing. If this has happened to you, you might find that kissing has become secondary in importance to the real objective, sexual intercourse. Starting to think about kissing as something pleasurable and desirable in itself will help you start to develop new relational frames about it.

Hugging/Rubbing

Hugging and rubbing, once commonly called petting, can take on new meanings if you can visualize them as viable forms of adult sexual expression. Hugging and rubbing, even with your clothes on, can be intensely pleasurable and can be carried to the point of orgasm with no risk of pregnancy or disease. You probably heard these referred to as dry humping, a reference to keeping moist genitals away from each other, usually by keeping your clothes on.

An interesting way to discover the delights of dry humping is to take the dryness out of it and rub against your partner to the point of orgasm. It can actually provide powerful orgasms because you control the pace, pressure, and intensity of stimulation. Try spreading lotion on your partner's breasts, chest, or buttocks. Take your clothes off and rub your penis or vulva back and forth and up and down between your partner's breasts, chest, or buttocks until you come. If your mind tells you things like, "how childish this is. I am not 15 anymore. Why waste time doing this when I could be doing the real thing," step back and remind yourself that this is exactly the kind of outdated thinking that limits your sexual pleasure and contributes to getting stuck. There are many men and women who find it easier to have enjoyable sexual sensations and orgasms through this kind of controlled rubbing than through sexual intercourse. Why not think of this as just another way to have fun sexually with your partner instead of viewing it as something less than intercourse?

Massage

Massage is one of the greatest sensual delights you can share with your partner. It is an excellent way to show your gratitude towards your partner while building mindfulness. I will cover massage in detail in chapter 14. The focus will be on pleasing your partner by giving her a massage. See chapter 14 for more detail.

Masturbation

One of the activities that can link your sensuality to your sexuality is masturbation. I will be covering masturbation in detail in chapter 15. Once again the focus will be on pleasing your partner through masturbation. I give complete instructions on how to masturbate him or her. See chapter 15 for more details.

Oral Sex

Oral sex is one of the most intimate forms of sexual expression because it involves face-to-genital contact. In chapter 16 I'll focus on how to please your partner orally. I will give complete instructions for how to perform oral sex on your male or female partner. Once again, the emphasis will be on pleasing your partner and showing your gratitude. See chapter 16 for more details.

Sexual Intercourse

The term sexual intercourse implies that two different types of connections occur when two humans interact sexually: (1) there is a sexual connection and (2) there is an interpersonal one. I'll discuss both of these aspects in detail in Chapter 17 and describe how to enjoy sexual intercourse as a multicourse gourmet meal.

The purpose of reviewing this continuum of sexual activities was to expose you to a host of different ways to give and receive sexual pleasure. Each type of activity has distinct advantages and disadvantages that only you can assess for yourself. As you read about them, the thoughts, self-talk, emotions, and mental images that arise have their origin in relational frames about sex developed over the course of your lifetime. If you find yourself getting hooked by thinking traps or outdated thoughts and feelings that are no longer helpful, try to step back and distance yourself from these thoughts and become an observer of them rather than take them all literally. Remember—this is your mind telling you things about these behaviors that may or may not be helpful in meeting your current sexual relationship goals.

Now that you've read about the continuum of sexual behaviors it is time to start becoming more mindful of your thoughts, feelings, self-talk, and mental images about them. The following three exercises are designed to help you examine your sexual behavior from a variety of different perspectives. This will help you understand what your mind is telling you about your sexual activity and whether or not it is helping you and is consistent with your sexual values and relationship goals.

Sexual Behavior Exercise # 1: My Favorite Sexual Behaviors

Purpose: People engage in a variety of behaviors to satisfy their sexual wants and needs. The purpose of this activity is to explore in a nonjudgmental way exactly what turns you on.

Instructions:

1. Describe which solo sexual activity you find most enjoyable. If you do not engage in solo sexual activity, simply state this.
2. What do you find most pleasurable about this activity?
3. Which partnered sexual activity do you find most satisfying?
4. What do you find most pleasurable about this activity?
5. Describe your favorite sexual position and explain what you like about it.

6. Describe your favorite sexual fantasy. If you do not fantasize, simply state this.
7. Are your thoughts, self-talk, mental images, and emotions about your sexual behavior helpful or unhelpful in staying true to your sexual values and meeting your sexual relationship goals?
8. Consider sharing this information with your sex partner.

With the widespread availability of sex online the issue of cybersex is worth looking at. There are various forms of cybersex ranging from watching XXX video clips to masturbating while talking to a live person on the phone or on a sex cam. Cybersex can be a thorny issue in relationships and marriages where one partner feels it is no big deal and not cheating and the other does. Like our initial discussion in chapter one about oral sex, many people do not believe that cybersex is real sex because there is no physical contact between the participants. Others feel that it is a breach of the emotional or spiritual bond the couple shares. I'm going to leave this kind of decision-making to you.

Sexual Behavior Exercise # 2: Is Cybersex, Sex?

Purpose: People vary in their beliefs about cybersex. The purpose of this activity is to help you identify your beliefs about cybersex and how they relate to your being stuck in a sexual rut.

Instructions:

1. Re-read the section on autoeroticism in chapter 14.
2. Answer the following questions:

    - Is cybersex really sex?
    - Is it possible to have an affair with someone over the Internet?
    - Is it "cheating" to be sexually explicit with another person over the Internet or phone?

- Is it cheating to masturbate while engaging in Internet or telephone sex?
- What are the dangers associated with Internet chatting or telephone sex?

3. Are your thoughts, self-talk, mental images, and emotions about autoeroticism and cybersex helpful or unhelpful in staying true to your sexual values and meeting your sexual relationship goals?

Sexual Behavior Exercise # 3: Unfinished Sentences

Purpose: People sometimes have a hard time answering questions about their sexual wants and needs. The purpose of this activity is to use sentence stems to make this easier for you to do.

Instructions:

1. Finish the following sentence stems:

    - Regarding sex, I wish my partner...
    - The sexual thing I want the most from my partner is...
    - The sexual thing I'd love to do to my partner is...
    - If there is one thing I could change about my sexual relationship with my partner it would be...

2. Consider sharing this information with your partner.

Chapter 7

Your Sexual Response

If you ask the average person which body part is most important regarding their sexual response, they'll probably say, *the penis* or *the vagina* or something else related to their genitals. Most of us equate sexual response to genital functioning, something that goes on between our legs. In fact, the most important body part involved in your sexual response is located between your ears.

Your brain, not your genitals, is the seat of your sexual response. Sexual response begins and ends in your mind. Sexual response is a complex interaction of psychological and physiological factors that starts in your brain and spreads through the rest of your body, including your genitals (Blonna and Carter, 2018).

It Starts with Desire

Your sexual response starts with your mind's perception of desire. This involves thoughts about yourself, your partner, and the specific context in which your potential sexual encounter occurs. In other words, three variables are involved; you, your partner, and the time and place of the encounter.

Your thoughts, feelings, personal scripts, and mental images about yourself set the stage for how you respond sexually to your partner in any given context. If you feel good about yourself and have helpful self-talk and mental images, this fuels desire and your brain will initiate sexual arousal. If your mind is filled with troubling thoughts, painful emotions, and unhelpful self-talk and mental images, you'll have difficulty feeling desire and becoming aroused.

The same model can be applied to the way your mind thinks and feels about your partner and the context in which everything plays out.

If you think someone is sexy and you have helpful thoughts, feelings, self-talk, and mental images about the person you will feel desire and your body will start to turn on, regardless of what the person looks like, smells like, or whether they match up to some societal standard for beauty, sexiness, etc.

The context is important because when and where the potential sexual encounter occurs will influence what you think and how you feel about it. The same partner under the right circumstances is a turn-on. Under different circumstances that same person might not turn you on. In a nutshell, your sexual response is quite subjective because it starts with what your mind tells you about yourself and your partner based on your standards for sexiness.

As you can see, your past relational frames regarding these three variables exert an influence on the whole process. Your thoughts, emotions, personal scripts, and mental images about yourself, your partner, and the specific time and place can be either helpful or unhelpful in facilitating your sexual response. Furthermore, as you will see in later sections of this book, the *quality* of your sexual experience, whether you consider it satisfying or unsatisfying, is also influenced by what your mind tells you about it.

Sexual response is subjective and strongly influenced by what your mind tells you about the experience. The subjectivity of sexual response is one of the most interesting things about it. Things that turn you on and fuel your desire might turn off the person sitting next to you.

The Anatomy and Physiology of Desire

Let's use an example with Ben and Alyssa to help explain how the three variables work together in initiating sexual response. Imagine that Ben is a free-lance writer who works from home. Alyssa, his wife of seven years, is a realtor who works for a large real estate company. Both have very flexible schedules, and it isn't unusual for Alyssa to work from home or drop in on Ben unexpectedly during the day while he is writing.

Ben is working on his computer in the waterfront house he shares with Alyssa. As a writer, Ben spends most afternoons in his second floor office, watching the boats go by on the water as he works on his freelance writing projects. Alyssa is off trying to close a deal on a large, waterfront home in a neighboring town. Ben expects she will be gone most of the day, giving him some quiet time to finish a big project that's due early next week.

Ben has been working since early this morning, putting the finishing touches on a travel piece he is writing for a large hotel chain. His mind is fully involved in what he's doing. His fingers move quickly over the keyboard and his eyes are focused on the screen; his attention is centered on his work. As he works on his proposal, he's barely aware of Alyssa's car approaching and pulling into the driveway. He hears the garage door open and looks out the window just in time to catch a glimpse of Alyssa's long legs through the sunroof as she pulls her car into the garage.

As soon as this happens, Ben's brain notes Alyssa's jet black hair cascading down over her shoulders and onto the outline of her breasts. She is wearing one of his favorite charcoal grey business suits with a silky white blouse underneath. He loves the way the outfit hugs her curves and shows off her legs. Alyssa enters the house through the garage and calls up to him, "*Hi honey, I'm home a little early. Hope you don't mind. I've got some great news to share.*"

Ben replies, "*No problem, hon,*" and continues with his work. Although he can't see her yet, he hears her in the kitchen rummaging through the drawers while humming a song. Ben, momentarily distracted by the vision of Alyssa and the sound of her voice, finds himself beginning to get an erection. He chuckles to himself and refocuses his attention on his writing.

After about 20 minutes the house gets quiet, and Ben smells a trace of Alyssa's perfume coming through the open door to his office.

The smell of her perfume causes his mind to wander and once again he feels his body begin to respond, this time to the presence of her scent. He feels his penis begin to get erect and although he tries to fight it, his mind continues to wander, drifting from his writing to his erection, to thoughts of Alyssa's warm body and their past lovemaking. His brain is just about to shut down this sexual response again when he realizes that she has entered the room and is standing quietly by the door, an open bottle of champagne and two glasses in her hand.

Alyssa slowly enters the room and, with a sexy smile, wanders over to Ben's desk and says, *"I closed the sale. Want to celebrate?"* She takes his glasses off his nose, wraps her arms around his shoulders, and begins to nibble on his ear. Ben is about to burst the zipper on his pants. He turns, gives her a kiss, and feels his penis grow even bigger as his body responds to her warmth, softness, and perfumed delights.

After a few sips of champagne his desire continues to sweep over his body and mind. Ben decides to stop trying to fight his brain's urges and allows his body to take over. He picks up Alyssa, carries her over to the day bed in his office, and begins to tear his clothes off as fast as he can. They proceed to make love, both deciding that Ben's writing can wait for a while.

As you can see from this example, the three factors involved in the sexual encounter—Ben, his partner Alyssa, and the context, mid-day in their home—came together in perfect combination for Ben's mind and body to respond sexually. Maybe on a different day, when he was stressed out about having to make a deadline, Alyssa's desire for an intimate afternoon celebration would have been a turn-off. For sexual response to initiate and continue all three variables must come together in your mind in a helpful way.

The following activity, *Things That Turn Me On*, will help you begin to be more mindful of your sexual turn-ons and turn-offs. You can share this information with your partner to create a more satisfying sex life.

Sexual Response Exercise # 1: Things That Turn Me On

Purpose: We all have different things that fuel our desire. You can't assume that your partner knows and understands your turn-ons or you hers. This activity is designed to help you explore and share the things that start your desire burning.

Instructions:

1. Think about the sexual turn-ons and messages sent back and forth between Ben and Alyssa in the preceding section of this chapter.
2. Think about your own sexual response, the things that turn you on and off.
3. Describe your personal turn-ons and turn-offs for each category listed below. Although the case study involves heterosexuals, all people (straight, gay, bisexual, transgendered) respond the same way physiologically to sexual turn-ons.

Turn-Ons

Sights (image of a sexy partner)
Sounds (background sounds and/or partner sounds)
Tastes (food, drink, and/or your partner)
Touches (how and where you like to be touched and to touch your partner)
Smells (perfume, cologne, background and/or your partner)
Behavior (preliminaries that get the blood flowing)

Turn-Offs

Go through the above list substituting turn-offs.

4. Share these lists with your partner.
5. Do you and your partner respond to the same turn-ons and turn-offs? If not, how can you use this information to problem-solve and improve the quality of your sexual relationship?
6. Are your thoughts, self-talk, mental images, and emotions about your turn-ons helpful or unhelpful in becoming aroused when making love with your partner?

Sexy Brain Basics

Three major parts of your brain work together during sexual response: (1) your thinking brain (the cerebral cortex), (2) your feeling brain (the limbic system) and, (3) your switchboard (the Thalamus and Hypothalamus). The three parts work together with your nervous and endocrine systems to turn you on and fuel your sexual arousal (Blonna, Carter, Levitan, 2011). You probably also noticed from the example with Ben that initially he was able to consciously switch his desire on and off before finally giving in to his passion. Your mind has the power to switch your sexual response on and off when you want it to.

Your Thinking Brain: The Cerebral Cortex

The conscious awareness of sensations is controlled by your cerebral cortex, the thinking part of your brain. In the example used, you can see how sensations (sight, sound, smell, and touch) associated with Alyssa entered Ben's consciousness. He became aware of these sensations as they entered the thinking part of his brain through visual (sight), auditory (sound), olfactory (smell) and tactile (touch) sensory areas and were interpreted by his mind as sexual cues to a potential encounter with Alyssa. These were the initial triggers of his desire and arousal. As with Ben, the sensual pathway to sexual response is through your cerebral cortex.

Although each sensation entered as a distinct, separate entity (the sight of Alyssa, hearing her voice, smelling her perfume, etc.), they were quickly assimilated, sorted out, deciphered, and combined as a signal for a potential sexual encounter. All of this activity was related to Ben's past sexual relational frames. His thoughts, feelings, personal scripts and mental images of how things would play out with Alyssa in the present moment were all rooted in his past relational frames created over time with her. They were also connected to his values related to sex and his relationship with Alyssa. One of his goals throughout their marriage has been to strengthen their sexual relationship, a major source of pleasure and a bond between them.

Your Feeling Brain: The Limbic System

The limbic system is a complex arrangement of nerve tissue that links your emotional brain with your thinking brain. In this way, the limbic system establishes a relationship between your thoughts and your feelings. Sometimes this relationship is clear-cut and easy to understand, and other times it is not. Sometimes your sexual emotions get the better of you and you don't think clearly about possible sexual cues or encounters. You might interpret someone's verbal communication, body language, or behavior as conveying an interest in having sex when they aren't interested. These mixed sexual messages can initiate sexual response at inappropriate times.

Fortunately, your cerebral cortex has the ability to exert conscious control over this and shut down your sexual response at any point. This may result in some frustration and genital engorgement or *blue balls*, a term often used to describe this phenomenon in men. Unfortunately, there is no commonly accepted term to describe similar arousal and frustration in women. Perhaps, the term, *blue vulva* or *blue lips* captures this for women.

In Ben's case his feelings of love and lust for Alyssa began to take over as the thinking part of his brain struggled to maintain its rational commitment to finishing his work. His thoughts of Alyssa, how her body felt, how much he cared for her, how much he desired her, started a tug of war between his rational concerns for continuing to work and his sexual feelings for Alyssa. Eventually these feelings won out and he put his work on hold.

Your Switchboard: The Thalamus and Hypothalamus

The thalamus and hypothalamus form the central core of your brain and play a crucial role in the continuation of your sexual response that began with your interpretation of incoming sensations as sexual. Ben's switchboard allowed his body to continue to respond to Alyssa's presence. Once Ben's cerebral cortex felt desire, it triggered his thalamus and hypothalamus, two small organs nestled in the base of his brain to jump start the rest of his sexual response. They triggered chemical (hormones) and electrical (nerve transmissions) stimulation of his nervous and endocrine systems to activate all of the organs, glands and tissues involved in his sexual response cycle.

The Sexual Response Cycle

So far, you've seen with the example of Ben and Alyssa how your body and mind work together to get sexual response started. In this section I'll take you through the entire sexual response cycle from arousal, through orgasm, and back to the un-aroused state. Most of what is known about human sexual response comes from the groundbreaking work of Masters and Johnson. In 1996 they published their ground-breaking book, *Human Sexual Response* (Masters and Johnson, 1966).

The book was ground-breaking for several reasons. Although previous researchers (Kinsey being the most notable) had published studies concerning self-reported *sexual behavior*, Masters and Johnson's was the first large-scale study of *sexual response*. Masters and Johnson were the first researchers to conduct large-scale sexual response studies in a laboratory setting. They were the first mainstream scientists to apply the scientific rigor necessary to quantify and qualify a very private act. Their work provided a graphic depiction of the actual sexual processes involved in sexual activity. Masters and Johnson invented the technology, instrumentation, and methodology needed to study the most intimate of all human activity.

Masters and Johnson created a language of sexuality that among other things operationally defined the term orgasm. While this might not seem like such a big deal today, in 1966 it was a breakthrough for scientists interested in studying human sexuality. An operational definition was a prerequisite for legitimate experimental research related to sexual response.

In addition to defining orgasm, they also coined the terms vasocongestion (engorging of genitals with blood during sexual arousal), and myotonia (involuntary muscle contractions). The use of these and other sexual terms allowed professionals in the field to communicate with each other and disseminate their research findings.

Masters and Johnson were the first researchers to divide sexual response into four sequential phases. The phases were: (1) excitement, (2) plateau, (3), orgasm and (4) resolution. They found that this sequencing of sexual response was the same regardless of the nature of sexual stimulation (masturbation, intercourse, and so forth) or one's sexual orientation (heterosexual, homosexual, bisexual).

Excitement

Desire and arousal combine to form excitement, the first stage of the sexual response cycle. Desire is the mental component that triggers arousal, the physical part of excitement.

Excitement can be triggered by a limitless array of thoughts, feelings, personal scripts, and mental images. Two key processes are involved in the excitement phase—vasocongestion and myotonia. Vasocongestion is the process that causes the erectile tissue in your genitals to engorge with blood. Myotonia is the build-up of muscle tension throughout your body.

During vasocongestion, blood vessels in your genitals dilate (open up), resulting in increased blood flow to your genitals. The increased blood flow fills up the spongy tissue that makes up this region of your body. During vasocongestion the blood flow into your genitals is greater than outflow. As this tissue fills with blood, it becomes engorged, enlarging in size, deepening in color, and increasing in sensitivity. If you are a man, this causes your penis to get erect and your scrotum (balls) to darken in color. If you are a woman, this causes your labia (vaginal lips) and clitoris to swell and deepen in color, your vagina to start lubricating, and your breasts to enlarge and become more sensitive.

Myotonia is responsible for the gradual build-up of tension in your skeletal muscles. This gradual build-up of muscular tension is progressive and pleasurable and occurs throughout your entire body, including your genitals. If you are a man, muscle tension in your scrotum causes your testes to elevate and move closer to your body. If you are a woman, the inner two-thirds of your vagina expands and your uterus (womb) is pulled backward.

Plateau

During plateau, the second phase of the sexual response cycle, the processes that were set into motion during the excitement phase reach their maximum levels. You experience peak levels of genital engorgement, color changes, lubrication, and muscular tension. If you are a man you penis becomes fully erect, your testes become completely elevated, and a small gland near your prostate called the Cowper's gland releases clear, slippery, pre-ejaculatory fluid (pre-cum), signaling intense sexual arousal. You'll also experience a sex flush, a rash-like reddish tinge to the skin of your chest and back associated with dilation of the blood vessels and increased blood flow in these areas. If you are a woman, your labia and clitoris reach their maximum size, and your clitoris retracts under its protective hood at the top of your vaginal opening. You will also experience the same sex flush that a man would get.

Plateau is the most variable stage in the cycle in terms of time. In general, if you are older and more sexually experienced, you will be able to prolong the plateau phase if you want to. If you are younger and less sexually experienced you will probably have shorter plateau periods.

Orgasm

Orgasm, the third phase of the sexual response cycle, is characterized by the dramatic release of tension and a decrease in your heart rate, blood pressure, breathing rate and the other physiological processes associated with the excitement and plateau stages. During orgasm most of your sexual organs undergo rhythmic, muscular contractions. These are responsible for the pleasurable release of pent-up muscular tension that you feel. In addition, orgasm triggers ejaculation, the release of fluid that contains sperm (in men) and other liquids from your internal sexual organs.

Resolution

During resolution, the last phase of the sexual response cycle, your body returns to its un-aroused state. After you have an orgasm (or orgasms if you are a woman), the engorgement of your genital tissue with blood, and the build-up of muscle tension throughout your body begins to reverse. Orgasm triggers your brain to normalize the dilation and constriction of your blood vessels, your heart rate, and your blood pressure. This normalization process allows your blood flow to return to normal. If you are a man, this causes your erection to shrink and the color and size of your genitals to return to normal. If you are a woman, you will begin to stop lubricating and the color and size of your genitals and breasts will return to normal. In addition, the release of muscular tension and expenditure of energy results in a generalized relaxation response throughout your body.

Masters and Johnson coined the term *refractory period* to describe the time required after an orgasm before you could enter the excitement stage again. Masters and Johnson found tremendous variability in this time between men and women, and among individual men. They found that women did not have a refractory period. If you are a woman, you don't need time to recover from the effects of an orgasm to get excited again. You can continue to stay lubricated and achieve another orgasm without resting as long as you continue being stimulated and are interested in continuing.

If you are a man you will need a certain amount of down time before you can achieve another erection. The amount of time you'll need will vary depending upon your age and the time since your last orgasm. In general, the younger you are and the longer the time since your last orgasm, the shorter your refractory period will be. In other words, a younger man who hasn't had an orgasm in some time would become re-aroused much more quickly than an older man who recently had an orgasm. Other variables, such as your overall level of health, stress, and obesity, are also related to the length of your refractory period.

Since Masters and Johnson published their findings, other researchers have come up with different variations of the sexual response cycle. I'll go over a few of the major studies briefly.

Helen Singer Kaplan (1985) argued that Masters and Johnson's four-phase sexual cycle neglected the importance of sexual desire in human sexual response. Furthermore, she claimed that the plateau stage was indistinguishable from excitement and the two stages should be merged together. She developed a triphasic model of sexual response that included desire, excitement, and orgasm phases (Kaplan,

1985). She placed most of the emphasis on desire and the role of the brain in initiating sexual response.

Walen and Roth (1987) developed a cognitive model of human sexual response that emphasized the importance of perception and cognitive factors in the initiation and perpetuation of sexual response. They accepted most of Masters and Johnson's findings related to the physiology of sexual arousal but argued that a sexual stimulus is only erotic if you perceived it to be. Something that is capable of turning a person on sexually may not do so in all situations and under all circumstances. In other words, it is not just the sexual stimulus that creates the turn-on, your perception and acceptance of it are what allow your body to become sexually aroused.

William Stayton (2002) developed a model that provided a spiritual and theological perspective on sexual response and pleasure. Stayton believed that love, spirituality, and sexuality were inextricably bound together and that God created people who are sexual in the fullest sense of the word. Stayton's basic premise is that it is not by coincidence that sexual response was so pleasurable. He believed that God created humans in such a way as to respond to sexual pleasure. He cited Masters and Johnson's discovery of the clitoris as the center of sexual response in women as evidence that God intended humans to be sexual creatures, enjoy this blessing, and perpetuate the species.

Rosemary Basson (2000) developed a model that, like Walen and Roth's, emphasized the role played by cognitive factors in sexual response. She emphasized that positive thoughts and feelings such as trust, caring, and happiness about one's partner are necessary for intimacy to exist and sexual response to occur. Negative thoughts and feelings such as anger, fear, and unhappiness can sabotage intimacy and make desire and arousal difficult, if not impossible. She also proposed that men and women differ in their sexual response. Basson proposed that emotional factors and intimacy issues were central to understanding sexual response in women. She found that female sexual response does not begin with desire or arousal as it does in men—it begins with intimacy. For many women, the starting point for their sexual response is not the desire for sex (physical sexual release) but the desire for intimacy (being close emotionally and physically with one's partner).

A Quick Word About Sexual Hormones

The role of sex hormones in sexual response is confusing. Part of the confusion comes from labeling hormones as *male* or *female*. In fact, the primary *male hormone*, testosterone, and *female hormone,* estrogen, are similarly produced in both men and women in their adrenal glands.

Testosterone is the hormone that seems to exert the most dramatic effect on sexual response and is associated with desire in both men and women. Men produce more testosterone than women (6 - 8 mg vs. 0.5 mg daily). The majority of men's testosterone (about 95%) is manufactured in the testes, and the remainder is produced in the adrenal glands. Women manufacture their testosterone in their ovaries and their adrenal glands (Blonna and Carter, 2018).

Before reaching puberty, boys and girls have similar amounts of testosterone produced in their adrenal glands. After puberty, men begin to produce larger amounts of the hormone in their testes.

Although men produce much more testosterone than women daily, women need less of it to derive the erotic effects of this potent hormone. Deficiencies of this hormone result in a drop-off in sexual desire in both men and women. Men are especially dependent on testosterone levels for sexual performance. When testosterone levels drop, men have difficulty obtaining and maintaining erections. Women's sexual performance does not seem to be affected as much by testosterone levels. When their levels of testosterone drop, they may still be able to experience lubrication and orgasm, despite having low levels of desire.

Estrogen levels also are related to sexual response. Women manufacture estrogens in their ovaries, whereas men produce it in small amounts their testes. Estrogens play a role in maintaining vaginal lubrication, thus facilitating intercourse. Women who have had their ovaries removed through hysterectomy and other procedures do not experience a reduction in sexual *desire,* but may experience vaginal dryness due to reduced lubrication. Women with high levels of estrogen do not experience heightened (or reduced) levels of sexual desire. Men also do not seem to be affected by too little estrogen. Excessive estrogen in men can have a feminizing effect that includes breast enlargement and erectile difficulties (Blonna and Carter, 2018).

Your Mind and Your Sexual Response

Your sexual response begins with what your mind tells you about yourself, your partner, and your anticipation of the experience itself. As I mentioned earlier in the chapter, in order for your body to respond sexually you need to have the right mindset, be in the right setting, and be with the right partner. All three of these variables are influenced by your thoughts, feelings, self-talk, and mental images about them.

If you go back to the Ben and Alyssa's example you can see how this worked out. Nowhere in the dialogue was there troubling thoughts or emotions and negative self-talk. Ben did not berate himself or undermine his ability to be sexually receptive to Alyssa. He wasn't angry at her or worried about taking time off from his work. The picture he saw in his mind when he thought about Alyssa was pleasurable and loving. His thoughts, feelings, and self-talk about making love with her were helpful in triggering his sexual response.

If he was angry at her or worried about work, or if he doubted his ability to respond to her or had negative mental images about how the encounter would set back his work project or end up in an argument with Alyssa, these thoughts and feelings would have sabotaged his sexual response. Under these circumstances it would have been difficult for his mind to trigger the beginning of his sexual response.

Think about how your own thoughts, feelings, self-talk, and mental images came together during your last sexual encounter. How did they influence your ability to respond and the quality of your sexual experience? Did they facilitate what you were expecting or contribute to something else? The remainder of this book will examine how your thoughts, feelings, self-talk, and mental images influence your sexuality in all of its dimensions. It will continue to explore the link between these factors and your sexual response. It will also look at other aspects of your sexuality such as your picture of yourself as a man or woman (gender role), your body image, your sexual orientation, your sexual behavior, and your sexual relationships.

Part 2
Becoming More Mindful

Chapter 8

A Deep Dive Into Mindfulness

Humans are mindful creatures. As newborns, we establish a bond to our mothers and caregivers through our senses. We respond to a warm gentle touch. We develop a sense of security and trust as we are held, cuddled, have our diapers changed, and are swaddled in soft, warm clothing and bedding. Sounds become familiar and reassuring. We pay attention to soft encouraging words, soothing music, and natural background sounds. The sound of a bird at our window captures our attention as much as the reassuring words of a caring parent. We lock on to our mother's eyes as she breastfeeds us and our father's eyes as he gives us a bottle or carefully spoons baby food into our mouth and gently wipes the excess off of our chins. We not only taste our food, we experience it with our other senses. We follow the flight of mobiles, dust motes, shadows, and other visual delights as they enter our field of vision. We don't have to be taught to mindfully experience life in the present moment. We are born with the ability to do so.

This carries on into early childhood. A good example of this is how toddlers play in the grass. Watch toddlers play in the grass for a while. They roll around in it, close their eyes, lie back in it, and listen to the sounds the wind makes as it blows through the high blades. They pull out handfuls of grass, throw them up in the air, and watch the blades fall to earth. They take a blade of grass and examine it carefully, rolling it around in their fingers, maybe even against their cheeks with their eyes closed. As they squeeze the grass between their fingers, they notice that oils are secreted. They smell this oil and taste it. Satiated with the grass, they move on to the next activity.

What happens to our ability to experience life this mindfully as we grow into adults? How many adults take the time to experience grass like this anymore? What transforms the sensual, mindful child into the constrained adult? Do we feel that we have "been there, done that?" Are we too jaded to enjoy the simple, free, sensual delights that surround us? Are we too distracted or just too busy? Are we embarrassed to be seen playing in the grass?

Unfortunately, for most adults the answer to all of those questions is "yes." To a certain extent our busy lives get in the way. We spend our days getting ourselves ready for work, our kids ready for school, or our parents ready for adult day care. We suffer through long commutes to work, put in 8-10 hours on the job, and struggle through our return commutes. After work we rush to get the kids to their sports games, classes, or groups. We get mom or dad from day care and figure out what we are doing for dinner. Once everyone is back home, dinner is finished, and the mess is cleaned up, we collapse on the couch for a couple of hours of television before going to bed and doing it all again the next day. Managing this kind of hectic schedule makes it easy to rush through life and stop giving anything our full attention.

Despite the frantic pace and complexity of modern-day life, you can relearn how to slow down and regain that sensual connection to the world around you by practicing mindfulness. Through mindfulness training you can relearn what it means to be fully integrated in the present moment. It takes time and practice and a shift in mindset, but anyone can do it.

Mindfulness Defined

Mindfulness is a state of being. Mindfulness meditation and other awareness-building exercises are tools to help you achieve a mindful state. Germer et al, (2005) described mindfulness as a four-dimensional state of being. They describe mindful moments as being:

- present centered
- nonjudgmental
- nonconceptual
- silent

Mindful Moments are present centered. *Present centered* means that the focus of mindful moments is always the *present,* never the *past* or the *future.* Mindfulness training helps you become more aware of when your mind jumps back to something that has already happened or ahead to something that is going to happen in the future. It also teaches you how to be more accepting of this and then redirect your focus back to the present moment.

Mindful moments are not judgmental. During mindful moments you just *notice* what is going on in your mind or your environment. You don't *judge* or *evaluate* what you are experiencing, you just *accept* it for what it is. Accepting reality, however painful, is a hallmark of mentally healthy people.

Mindful moments are not thinking moments. There is a difference between just noticing and *thinking.* Thinking moments involve planning, figuring things out, sorting things out and solving problems. Planning, figuring out, sorting out, and solving problems takes you *out* of just noticing the present moment. Mindfulness training helps you become more aware of those moments when your mind goes beyond just noticing and gets into planning, figuring out, sorting, or problem.

Mindful moments are always silent moments. Whenever you add speech to a mindful moment you take it to a different conceptual level that takes you out of just noticing and into higher level thinking. The talking that goes on during mindful moments is *self-talk,* also known as *sub-vocal speech.* Mindful self-talk revolves around noticing, labeling, and accepting images, thoughts, feelings, sounds, body sensations etc. in the present moment.

Let me give you a sexual example and show you how this plays out regarding making love with your partner. Imagine that you are making love with your partner. If you were doing it mindfully here is what would be going on:

Present Centered—You would be fully attentive to what is going on with your partner. You would be experiencing your partner with all five senses. Your thoughts would only focus on what is going on with your two bodies as you make love. They would not drift to something that happened yesterday or will happen tomorrow.

Nonconceptual—Instead of thinking about why things are going the way they are you would simply note what is happening and enjoy it. You wouldn't be trying to figure out or anticipate anything. You would accept your sexual experience for what it is and allow it to play out however it does.

Nonjudgmental—You wouldn't judge or compare your partner and your lovemaking to anything. You would enjoy and accept your partner and your lovemaking for what it is, not for what it could be or should be according to some societal standard.

Nonverbal—You wouldn't be talking a lot. You would communicate what had to be said with your body and your spirit.

Imagine what you sex life would be like if you could approach each sexual experience in such a mindful way. Obviously, there are times when looking to the past or future, thinking, judging, and speaking all make sense and are the right things to do. However, when trying to un-clutter your mind and practice mindfulness, they interfere with the process. Don't worry if this is hard to accept at this point in your mindfulness training. This is where you need to just accept your confusion and discomfort and continue practicing.

The Practice of Mindfulness

As I mentioned in the Forward to this book, humans are born mindful. Even though we often lapse into mindlessness, we retain the ability to relearn what it means to be mindful and experience life in the present moment with all five senses. Practicing mindfulness revolves around two types of training, *formal* and *informal.* Each uses different activities to help you increase your attention to the present moment (Blonna, 2010).

Formal mindfulness training is a structured program of daily meditation practice. There are countless ways to teach people how to meditate. I teach mindfulness meditation in three steps:

- Diaphragmatic Breathing Training
- Breath Meditation Training
- Mindfulness Meditation Training

I find that breaking formal training down this way makes it easier for most people to relearn what it means to be mindful. In this non-threatening way you learn about the breath first, then apply that knowledge to learning how to meditate while focusing on the breath. Lastly, it sets the stage for learning mindfulness meditation. Starting beginners with mindfulness meditation is a sure-fire prescription for failure. It is simply too difficult for most people to jump right into mindfulness meditation practice and succeed.

Informal mindfulness training revolves around using simple exercises and activities that encourage you to be more mindful in everyday experiences. These exercises and activities are tailored to your daily behaviors and environments so they fit right into your lifestyle and personality. Informal mindfulness training involves learning how to devote your full attention to every activity you are engaged in.

Both formal and informal mindfulness training uses exercises and activities that focus on the internal and external environments. Your internal environment relates to your body and mind. This environment includes your thoughts, self-talk, mental images, and feelings. It also includes all body sensations. Your external environment relates to your behavior and physical surroundings. Becoming more aware of your external environment revolves around increasing your awareness of your behavior and what's going on in your immediate physical surroundings.

The two types of training and different environmental focus reinforce each other. For example, while practicing mindfulness meditation (a formal activity) you are aware of things going on in both your internal and external environments. You notice your thoughts, feelings and body sensations in addition to the sights, sounds, and smells of your physical environment. The increased awareness you develop practicing meditation help you when performing informal mindfulness activities such as mindful eating.

Let me give you a personal example using my morning routine. Every Tuesday, Thursday, and Saturday I set my alarm for 5:00am in order to get to the beach at sunrise to run and meditate. I bicycle down to the beach, an informal mindfulness activity, and spread out my blanket about 20 yards from the shoreline. I stretch and then go for a three-mile run.

I practice Breath Meditation, a formal mindfulness activity, while I run. I synchronize my breathing and footfalls as the focal point of my attention. For example, I might take four strides to inhale and four strides to exhale. I usually say to myself "*one, two, three, four*" as I inhale and repeat these words as I exhale. Whenever my thoughts drift from the words *one, two, three, four,* I redirect them back to my breathing and self-talk. As I run I am fully aware of the sights, sounds, smells, and climate of the beach. I do not shut these out but I do not focus on them.

When I finish my run I take off my shoes, grab a quick drink, and then float on my back in the surf for a few minutes to cool off. I use this time to practice *mindful floating*, an informal mindfulness activity. My awareness includes the sensations of floating and movement on my body, the warmth of the rising sun, the breeze blowing over me or the absence of a breeze. I gaze up at the sky and notice the clouds, the colors as they change, and any birds flying by.

After a few minutes I get out of the water, towel off, and start my sitting mindfulness meditation. I set my timer for 20 minutes, get comfortable by scooping out a place for my legs and gently building up the sand beneath my buttocks for a little elevation. I then focus on my breathing for a few moments before settling in and meditating with my eyes open. I usually focus on the horizon where the water meets the sky, but after several minutes I shift my focus to the waves breaking on the shoreline or the sand in front of my blanket. I take in all of the sights (including people walking by and birds flying by), sounds, smells, and sensations associated with the beach at sunrise. My mind simply notices, labels, and accepts these inputs into my consciousness. Whenever my mind strays to the past or the future I bring it back to the present by focusing on my breathing for a few moments. When my timer goes off I relax and enjoy the beach for a few moments before bicycling home again.

I love this schedule because it incorporates both formal and informal mindfulness practice using many of the things I value deeply and that make me happy. It combines my love of the early morning, sunrise, the beach, the gulf waters, running, meditating, and bicycling. I couldn't think of a better format for my meditation practice.

The Purpose of Mindfulness

Now that you understand what mindfulness is and how to become more mindful, you might ask yourself, why bother? I really want you to think about this because most people who don't follow through with their mindfulness training do so because they never really thought about why they wanted to start in the first place. People generally explore mindfulness for two main reasons: (1) to help them relax and manage stress, and (2) to enhance their spirituality, particularly their curiosity about Buddhism.

Using Mindfulness to Relax and Manage Stress

The Mindfulness Based Stress Reduction Program developed at Harvard over 40 years ago was one of the first programs that applied the principles and practices of mindfulness to helping people reduce their stress (Kabat-Zinn, 2013). Since then, hundreds of other mindfulness-based programs around the world have shown how mindfulness can help people manage a variety of issues in addition to stress. Mindfulness has also been incorporated into a variety of psychotherapeutic approaches to problems ranging from anxiety and depression to post-traumatic stress disorder.

Mindfulness-based programs have been shown to:

- improve overall mental health (less stress, fear, worry, anxiety, depression)
- improve overall physical health (mostly reduced cardiovascular risks, lower blood pressure, less anger and hostility)
- improve cognitive functioning (slow down runaway thinking paving the way for clearer, more reasoned thinking; improve ability to focus on one issue with full attention)
- enhance quality of relationships (greater awareness and appreciation of others, better listening, calmer responding)
- enhance appreciation of one's life (greater acceptance of one's position in life, fewer cravings etc.) (Germer, 2005).

Enhancing Spirituality

People often used the terms spirituality, faith and religion to refer to the same thing, a sense of being connected to something greater than the self. Although all three terms are related, they are very different.

Faith is the belief in something that cannot be proved empirically. Faith is really the bedrock of both spirituality and religion, yet you can have faith (in the self, for instance) and be neither spiritual nor religious.

Spirituality is defined as a sense of interconnectedness with a power greater than the self. This can't be proven empirically so if you are a spiritual person you also have faith. While spirituality is a cornerstone of religious participation and church membership, you can be spiritual and not be religious. Your sense of interconnectedness may be with the natural world or all human beings and not manifest itself in church membership.

Religion is an organized system of worship and belief. It includes faith and spirituality, but goes beyond them by institutionalizing them. Each religion has its own interpretation of, guidelines for, and rules regarding specific issues of faith and spirituality. While all religions incorporate faith and spirituality, each has a different theological perspective. Mindfulness meditation is the key tool used by Buddhists and others to deepen their spirituality. Practicing mindfulness meditation helps Buddhists stay focused on leading a life that revolves around the Eightfold Path and the Four Noble Truths. Like the Ten Commandments or other spiritual documents, the Eightfold Path and the Four Noble Truths provide guidelines for behavior that help Buddhists live a moral life in their spiritual path to nirvana. Mindfulness meditation was designed as the primary tool for increasing awareness of thoughts, feelings, and behaviors that are inconsistent with the Eightfold Path and the Four Noble Truths. When Buddhists "just sit" it is to develop awareness and acceptance of their lives in relation to these spiritual guidelines (Nathan, 1990).

Sex as Transcendence

Whether you believe that your *spirituality* connects you with God, some higher power, or all other living things, *transcendence* of the self is the key to spirituality. You've probably heard people describe orgasm in terms of feeling "uplifted," "out of this world," or "at one with the universe." I believe the transcendence that orgasm offers is inherent in our sexual response. I also believe that sex and orgasm with someone you love and are committed to gives you a heightened level of spirituality. Sharing an intense orgasm with your partner can, at times, make you feel instantly at one with the universe. If one positive human experience is capable of linking all of us together, it just might be orgasm.

Humans and other animals seem to share the ability to respond sexually to one another. Sexual activity with a partner, by its nature, connects us to someone else in a unique way. A high level of spiritual wellness can help us form sexual relationships based on caring and mutual respect, instead of exploitation and disrespect. Practicing sexual mindfulness contributes to building high-level spiritual wellness.

Chapter 9

Formal Mindfulness Training

Formal mindfulness training involves the regular practice of mindfulness meditation. To someone who has never meditated before this is a pretty daunting prospect. Because of this I ease students and clients into it in three stages:

- diaphragmatic breathing training
- breath meditation training
- mindfulness meditation training

I have found this approach works because it is incremental in terms of time and focus. For example, you can practice diaphragmatic breathing anywhere, even driving. As little as a few good breaths will help re-direct your focus and make you feel better. To practice either breath meditation or mindfulness meditation you need at least twenty minutes of uninterrupted time and a quiet location free from distractions. Breath meditation uses your breathing as the focal point of your mindfulness. It is more focused and of longer duration than diaphragmatic breathing, but easier than mindfulness meditation. True mindfulness meditation has no single focal point and instead focuses on the endless series of thoughts, feelings, images, and sensations. It starts with focusing on the breath to get centered, but then opens the doors of perception well beyond breathing. For at least twenty minutes you notice the activity of your body, mind, and environment without judgment. When your mind drifts back into the past or jumps into the future you bring your focus back to the present and what is going on in your body, mind, and environment.

Diaphragmatic Breathing

When I teach mindfulness meditation to my students and clients I always start by having them practice diaphragmatic breathing. Breathing is the basis of both life and all relaxation activities. One of the great ironies of breathing is how important it is, yet how little *attention* we pay to it. Although breathing is our biological and spiritual connection to the universe we usually take it completely for granted. In a sense, every time you breathe you recycle the very elements of life. You breathe in life-giving oxygen and recycle this back into the universe by exhaling carbon dioxide. This cycling of breath in and breath out is your connection to the universe and the cycle of life you share with other living things such as the trees and animals around you. Your breathing is also a spiritual process, as this cycle illustrates your interconnectedness to all living things on the planet and the universe beyond.

The simple practice of being more mindful of your breathing can help you get focused and back to the present moment. It can also be used to reduce your stress. When you practice mindful breathing your thinking slows down. Mindful breathing helps you stop overthinking, especially about past and future worries. The parts of your brain that control breathing are intimately related to the parts that control the stress response. Controlled, deep, even breathing facilitates relaxation. Rapid, shallow, irregular breathing disrupts relaxation. One of the main cues for understanding whether you are stressed is the pace and depth of your breathing. If it is rapid and shallow, chances are that you are stressed.

Learning to control your breathing will provide immediate benefits in learning to control your stress response. By breathing correctly you can strengthen and train your lung functioning, increase your cardiovascular response, increase oxygenation of your blood, calm your nerves, and increase restfulness. It also sets the stage for learning breath meditation.

Most of us use only a portion of our lungs when we breathe. We tend to breathe with the top third of the lungs. To receive the calming benefits of diaphragmatic breathing, you must learn how to get your entire lung capacity involved. You need to learn how to fill your lungs completely from the bottom up. Learning how to breathe this way takes practice but you can master it if you spend time each day doing so. I've found that knowing a little about the lungs and how the diaphragm works will help you master these two activities.

A Short Overview of the Diaphragm and Breathing

The diaphragm is a large band of muscle tissue that is attached all around the lower portion of your rib cage. It separates the contents of your chest cavity (the lungs, heart, etc.) from the contents of your abdominal cavity (stomach, intestines, etc.). Contracting and relaxing the diaphragm affects the volume of your chest cavity and the air pressure in your lungs.

When you breathe in, your diaphragm contracts and pulls downward, increasing the volume of your chest cavity and allowing air from outside your body to flow in. If you put your hands on your belly, just below your rib cage, when you breathe you can feel your belly push out as your diaphragm contracts and pulls downward. Some people call diaphragmatic breathing *belly breathing* because of this phenomenon. When you breathe out, your diaphragm relaxes, gets looser, and moves back to its normal position higher in your chest.

When you are stressed, the muscles in your abdomen tighten up and work against your diaphragm's natural downward push. This keeps the diaphragm from fully contracting and allowing maximum air to enter your lungs. One of the goals of diaphragmatic breathing is to help you relax your belly so you can deepen your breathing and get more life-giving air into your lungs. Remember: a hallmark of relaxation is a slow, deep, even breathing pattern. Regular practice of diaphragmatic breathing and diaphragmatic breathing meditation will help facilitate this.

The following exercise, *Diaphragmatic Breathing*, is designed to teach you how to perform diaphragmatic breathing. You can use diaphragmatic breathing by itself to put your body into a relaxed state and short-circuit the stress response. It also sets the stage for breath meditation and mindfulness meditation.

Formal Mindfulness Training Exercise # 1: Diaphragmatic Breathing

Instructions: To practice, simply follow the instructions below. You might find it easier to record these instructions and then listen to the recording.

1. Focus your attention on your current breathing pattern.
2. Make a mental note of the depth, pace, and regularity of your breathing.
3. Visualize a picture of your lungs and your diaphragm.
4. Slowly breathe in through your nose.
5. Rest your hands on your belly, just under your ribs.
6. Feel your belly move out as your diaphragm pushes down against it.
7. As you breathe in through your nose, visualize your lungs inflating completely, starting from the bottom (the part closest to your diaphragm) and moving upward.
8. Let your ribs expand and shoulders gently rise as your lungs inflate.
9. When you have filled your lungs, slowly exhale through your nose.
10. Feel your belly push back and your diaphragm rise back into place.
11. As you feel the movements in your belly, visualize your lungs emptying.

12. Imagine all of the air leaving your lungs as they deflate. (Sometimes, visualizing a balloon losing air or a toothpaste tube squeezing the paste out can be helpful in understanding the emptying process.)
13. Continue to breathe in and out this way for a couple of minutes, paying attention to the movement of your belly and diaphragm and the visual picture of your lungs filling from the bottom up and then completely emptying.

A Few Hints About Practicing Diaphragmatic Breathing:

Don't:

- Worry about the depth and pace of your breathing.
- Judge your performance.
- Compare yourself to people who have been meditating for years.
- Expect instant results. Give it time.

Do:

- Pay attention to what is going on in your lungs and the rest of your body.
- Accept that you will lose your focus during your practice.
- Accept that your runaway mind will need to be re-directed back to your breathing.
- Give yourself time to adjust to this new practice.

I have been practicing diaphragmatic breathing and breath meditation for over thirty years and I still get distracted. Some days it seems that my mind is all over the place. Other days I easily and gracefully fall into a deep state of relaxation and my mind is calm. I've learned to accept this and co-exist with my discomfort related to my runaway mind.

Relax. It will take time and practice to feel fully comfortable doing diaphragmatic breathing. As you become more comfortable with the practice you will be able to switch into this type of breathing on demand whenever you feel stressed. This is a very valuable first line of defense against stress when you find yourself in potentially stressful situations.

Breath Meditation

After a week of practicing diaphragmatic breathing I find that most people are comfortable enough with their breathing to use it as a focal point for meditating. When you are able to sit and do diaphragmatic breathing with your eyes open or closed for five minutes, you are ready to transform this into a meditative experience.

Diaphragmatic breath meditation involves noticing and paying full attention to your breath and what is going on in your diaphragm, lungs, and chest as you breathe in and out. When you get distracted from this you simply return your focus to what is going on in your diaphragm, lungs, and chest as you breathe in and out.

Formal Mindfulness Training Exercise # 2: Breath Meditation

Instructions: To practice, simply follow the instructions below. You might find it easier to record the instructions and then listen to the recording.

Instructions (Indoors):

1. Prepare to spend 5-30 minutes of uninterrupted activity where you will not be disturbed by other people, the doorbell, the telephone or anything else.

2. Wear comfortable clothing such as a sweat suit with a non-binding waistband.
3. Remove your shoes or sneakers.
4. Set the temperature in the room at a comfortable level, neither too hot nor too cold.
5. Set a timer to let you know when your time is up. Start with five minutes for the first week's practice. Add a minute each week until you can just sit for thirty minutes.
6. If you are sitting on the ground:

   - Spread a blanket or mat and place your cushion on it.
   - Sit on a cushion that raises your buttocks off the ground slightly and allows your legs to be slightly below you.
   - Cross your legs and pull one foot up over the other leg and rest it on your thigh or calf. This is known as the Half-Lotus Position. If you cannot do this simply cross your legs in a comfortable manner.
   - Sit up straight with your head, neck, and back in alignment. This is referred to as the Noble Posture and is important for proper breathing.
   - Take your time and readjust your legs, butt, back, and any other body part to get into a comfortable Noble Posture with your legs folded under you and your back, neck, and head in alignment.
   - Do not slouch. Readjust your position if you notice that you are slouching.
   - Fold your hands and let them rest comfortably on your lap or let each hand rest on a knee, palms facing up.
7. If you are sitting on a chair:

   - Take your shoes and socks off.
   - Keep your legs uncrossed with your feet resting comfortably on the floor.

- Sit up straight with your head, neck, and back in the Noble Posture.
- Take your time and readjust your legs, butt, back, and any other body part to get into a comfortable Noble Posture with your feet flat on the ground, with your back, neck, and head in alignment.
- Do not slouch. Readjust your position if you notice that you are slouching.
- Fold your hands and let them rest gently on your lap.

8. Focus your attention on your current breathing pattern.
9. Make a mental note of the depth, pace, and regularity of your breathing.
10. Visualize a picture of your lungs and your diaphragm.
11. Slowly breathe in through your nose.
12. Feel your belly move out as your diaphragm pushes down against it.
13. As you breathe in through your nose, visualize your lungs inflating completely starting from the bottom (the part closest to your diaphragm) and moving upward.
14. Let your ribs expand and shoulders gently rise as your lungs inflate.
15. When you have filled your lungs, slowly exhale through your nose.
16. Feel your belly push back and your diaphragm rise back into place.
17. As you feel the movements in your belly, visualize your lungs emptying.
18. Imagine all of the air leaving your lungs as they deflate. (Sometimes visualizing a balloon losing air or a toothpaste tube squeezing the paste out can be helpful in understanding the emptying process.)
19. As you continue to breathe in and out this way, pay attention to your thoughts. Try to keep your thoughts focused on your

breathing. You might find that saying "in" as you inhale and "out" as you exhale makes it easier to keep your focus on your breathing. Say these words to yourself. Some people find that counting the seconds it takes to inhale and exhale keeps them focused on their breathing.

20. Your mind will wander throughout your session. This is normal and still happens to veteran meditators.
21. When your thoughts stray from the present moment, do not get upset at yourself. Instead, tell yourself:

    - *My mind is taking me out of the here and now and into the* [wherever it's taking you].

22. If you find yourself evaluating or judging something, tell yourself:

    - *My mind is judging or evaluating again instead of merely noting* [whatever it's judging or evaluating].

23. If you find that you are getting angry at yourself, notice this and say:

    - *It is normal to get angry and frustrated at myself when my mind wanders. It is ok for me to do this.*

24. When your thoughts or feelings take you out of the present moment to the past or future:

    - Notice and accept the thoughts or feeling.
    - Acknowledge that it has taken you out of the present moment.
    - Shift your focus off the thoughts or feelings and back onto your breathing.
    - Close your eyes and return to focusing on your breathing for a few breaths.

25. Open your eyes and continue meditating until your timer goes off.
26. At the end of your session, come back to the present, open your eyes, and start to sit up and return to your day.

Practice at least three times a week, slowly increasing your time from five to thirty minutes. With a few months' practice, you will find that you can slow your breathing down and stay focused on it most of the time. Be patient and forgiving with yourself as you practice mindfulness meditation. It will take time and practice to get comfortable with it, but it is time well spent.

Mindfulness Meditation (Just Sitting)

Mindfulness meditation is often referred to as *Just Sitting.* The just sitting reference is both very descriptive and very misleading. In one sense, all you do when you perform mindfulness meditation is "just sit" for an extended period of time. This sounds pretty simple, direct, and uncomplicated. However, unlike other times when you just sit, during mindfulness meditation you not only sit, you also pay full attention to everything going on inside and outside your body and mind, as well as in the environment around you (Nathan, 1990; Kora, 1995).

In other words, you're fully aware of all of your thoughts, self-talk, mental images, and emotions. You're also fully aware of the sensations going on in your body. These might be related to muscle tension, pain, breathing, or any other physiological activities that you sense. In addition, you're aware of things going on around you. You're aware of the temperature and movement of air, sounds, scents, and anything else emanating from your environment. Your experience is 100 percent focused on the here and now and your internal and external environments.

Mindfulness meditation is similar to breath meditation, but differs in a few key ways. Unlike Breath Meditation, which is designed to relax your body and mind, Mindfulness Meditation is designed to increase your awareness of what is going on. Mindfulness Meditation uses your breath as a focal point, but only when your mind wanders out of the present moment and into the past or future. It also uses your breath as a tool to return to the present moment when you become aware that your mind is judging, comparing, problem-solving or doing something other than just noticing and accepting. During Mindfulness Meditation there is no attempt to censor your incoming thoughts, sounds, and other stimuli as long as they are related to the present.

Many people are frustrated when they initially learn how to perform mindfulness meditation because their focus is constantly interrupted by competing thoughts, feelings, and external stimuli. When they become aware of these distractions they react emotionally, becoming upset with themselves for allowing the distraction.

Rather than ignoring, suppressing, or evaluating these disruptions and thus getting emotionally involved with them, it is better to just note their presence, accept them, and continue to meditate. A key to understanding mindfulness meditation is realizing that it is based on developing an accepting attitude toward reality. The idea is to observe reality in a noncritical way.

This sounds simple, but is very hard to do. We are used to filtering our thoughts and feelings through a layer of experience and a list of shoulds, oughts, and musts (how things should, ought to, and must be) rather than seeing them the way they actually are.

To better understand how to deal with your mind wandering, let's imagine you are practicing mindfulness meditation. You are comfortably dressed, sitting quietly on an exercise mat, legs gently crossed, hands folded and gently resting in your lap. You've taken a few deep diaphragmatic breaths and are starting to pay attention to your thoughts and feelings and the sensations in your body and all around you. As you do this, you start thinking about a work project that is due tomorrow (thinking ahead instead of paying attention to the present). You start an inner dialogue with yourself and tell yourself, "I better remember to get my presentation checked tonight. It has got to be perfect for tomorrow's meeting." The next thing you are aware of is an emotional response. You start to criticize yourself for not finishing before you left work: "I'm such a jerk for not finishing the presentation. All I had to do was check it one last time." You continue by saying, "I'm probably going to do really poorly on the presentation because of this."

At this point you realize that your thoughts and emotions drifted from the present, back to the past, and into the future. To correct this you would simply note that this happened, accept it without being judgmental, and get back to paying attention to the present moment. Rather than continuing with this self-critical debate about your work habits, you simply tell yourself, "How interesting. Here I am having this debate about the presentation. When I am done meditating, I'll start thinking about it more." After this happens you get back to paying attention to the present moment and resume meditating until your session is over. Eventually, with practice and time, you become more proficient at staying focused, and it becomes easier to note the distractions in a nonjudgmental way and get back to paying full attention to the present moment.

Formal Mindfulness Training Exercise # 3: Just Sitting

You can meditate indoors or outdoors. I prefer to practice breath meditation indoors and mindfulness meditation outdoors. I find it easier to concentrate on my breathing when I am indoors because I can control the noise level, distractions, temperature, and visual stimuli. I can choose a quiet place in my home where I can close the shades, put the fan on slow, and sit on the floor in almost absolute silence. I almost always practice breath meditation with my eyes closed.

On the other hand I prefer to practice mindfulness meditation outdoors, usually at sunrise on the beach near my home. Since mindfulness meditation does not filter out any sights, sounds, smells, or sensations, I find the beach an exotic location for practice. I usually get down to the beach, find a nice place close to the shore where I can hear and see the waves, and scoop out a well for my legs and build a slight platform with the sand for my butt. I then cover the area with my blanket. I go for a three-mile run, float in the Gulf of Mexico for a few minutes to cool off, and then settle in on my blanket to meditate. I keep my eyes open and fix my vision on the waves, the horizon, or an area three to six feet in front of my blanket. I usually shift to these different focal points during the course of my meditation or close my eyes and focus on my breath if I get too distracted.

Since I already gave you directions for the indoor practice of breath meditation I will give you instructions for the outdoor practice of mindfulness meditation.

Instructions (Outdoors): To practice, simply follow the instructions below. You might find it easier to record the instructions and then listen to the recording.

1. Prepare to spend five to 30 minutes minutes of uninterrupted activity where you will not be disturbed by other people, your cell phone, or anything else.
2. Wear comfortable clothing, such as a sweat suit with a non-binding waistband.

    - The weather and location will determine this to a certain extent.
    - I almost always meditate barefoot and in a bathing suit since I meditate on the beach.

- If you are in a private place you may choose to go without clothes.

3. Remove your shoes or sneakers.
4. Set a timer to let you know when your time is up. Start with five minutes for the first week's practice. Add a minute each week until you can just sit for thirty minutes.
5. I recommend sitting on the ground when meditating outdoors, but if this is uncomfortable use the chair instructions.
6. If you are on the ground:

    - Spread a blanket or mat and place your cushion on it.
    - Sit on a cushion that raises your buttocks off the ground slightly and allows your legs to be slightly below you.
    - If you meditate on the beach, scoop out a depression for your legs to drop into. Use the sand to make a comfortable "seat" in front of the scooped-out area. Spread your blanket over this spot.
    - Cross your legs and pull one foot up over the other leg and rest it on your thigh or calf. This is known as the Half-Lotus Position. If you cannot do this simply cross your legs in a comfortable manner.
    - Sit up straight with your head, neck, and back in alignment. This is referred to as the Noble Posture and is important for proper breathing.
    - Take your time and readjust your legs, butt, back, and any other body part to get into a comfortable Noble Posture with your legs folded under you and your back, neck, and head in alignment.
    - Do not slouch. Readjust your position if you notice that you are slouching.
    - Fold your hands and let them rest comfortably on your lap or let each hand rest on a knee, palms facing up.

7. If you sit on a chair:

    - Take your shoes and socks off.
    - Keep your legs uncrossed with your feet resting comfortably on the floor.
    - Sit up straight with your head, neck, and back in the Noble Posture.
    - Take your time and readjust your legs, butt, back, and any other body part to get into a comfortable Noble Posture with your feet flat on the ground and your back, neck, and head in alignment.
    - Do not slouch. Readjust your position if you notice that you are slouching.
    - Fold your hands and let them rest gently on your lap.

8. Start by focusing your attention on your breathing. Unlike in breath meditation, do not attempt to regulate or control your breathing.
9. Close your eyes and notice the depth, pace, and regularity of your breathing.
10. Continue to notice the depth, pace, and regularity of your breathing for several breaths.
11. With your eyes either open or closed, begin to notice what goes on with the muscles and bones in your chest, abdomen, shoulders and neck as you breathe in and out.
12. Feel the air enter and exit your lungs.
13. Feel your chest muscles expand and contract and your shoulders rise and fall as you breathe.
14. Notice what happens in your neck and head as you breathe in and out. If you have disc issues in your neck and back, it is not unusual for you to hear and feel them pop as you focus on them.
15. Continue to breathe for several more breaths and notice what goes on with the muscles and bones in your chest, abdomen, shoulders and neck as you breathe in and out.

16. Open your eyes and choose a focal point in the area near you or off into the horizon.
17. Continue to breathe normally as you focus your attention on the area you have chosen.
18. Spend several moments noticing the details of what you are focusing on.

    - Notice the color, shape, size, patterns, etc. of the object(s) in your visual field.
    - Do not judge or compare what you are seeing.
    - Do not try to figure out why they look the way they do. Just accept them.

19. As you gaze out on your focal point, pay attention to the sounds in your immediate environment.

    - Try to isolate individual sounds and enjoy them.
    - Don't try to label or categorize them or worry about not knowing their origin.
    - Enjoy the sounds for what they are.

20. Now shift your focus to the other sensations in your environment.

    - Notice the temperature and feeling of warmth or coldness as they waft over your body.
    - Notice the movement of air—the volume, direction, and intensity of air flow.
    - Notice any smells entering your consciousness.
    - Don't judge them, just notice them.

21. Close your eyes and repeat steps 19 and 20.

    - Take several moments to notice the sounds, smells, and feelings associated with the movement of air in your environment.

22. Keep your eyes closed and shift your focus off the sensations in your outside environment and onto what is going on in your body.

    - Feel the sensations of warmth and relaxation in your body.
    - Refocus on your posture and be sure to sit straight without slouching.
    - Identify areas of muscle tension or pain. Try to sit with the tension and pain for a while and just accept it rather than fidget or readjust if you don't have to.
    - Notice things like perspiration and the effects of air movement on it.

23. Spend several moments focusing on your body with your eyes closed.
24. Open your eyes and spend the rest of your time breathing normally and focusing on the horizon or an object in your near environment.
25. Your mind will wander throughout your session. This is normal and still happens to veteran meditators.
26. When your thoughts stray from the present moment, do not get upset at yourself. Instead, tell yourself:

    - *My mind is taking me out of the here and now and into the* [wherever it's taking you].

27. If you find yourself evaluating or judging something, tell yourself:

    - *My mind is judging or evaluating again instead of merely noting* [whatever it's judging or evaluating].

28. If you find that you are getting angry at yourself, notice this and say:

- *It is normal to get angry and frustrated at myself when my mind wanders. It is ok for me to do this.*

29. If your anger, frustration, or any emotion takes you out of the present moment to the past or future, treat the emotion like you would a thought or mental image.

    - Shift your focus off the emotion.
    - Close your eyes and return to focusing on your breathing for a few breaths.

This will help you return to the present moment.

30. Open your eyes and continue meditating until your timer goes off.

Practice at least three times a week, slowly increasing your time from five to thirty minutes. With a few months' practice you will find that you can slow your breathing down and stay focused on it most of the time. Be patient and forgiving with yourself as you practice mindfulness meditation. It will take time and practice to get comfortable with it, but it is time well spent.

CHAPTER 10

Informal Mindfulness Training

Focus on the Internal Environment

As mentioned previously, informal mindfulness training activities focus on both your internal and external environments. Mindfulness training that focuses on your internal environment will help you become more aware of your thoughts, self-talk, mental images, and emotions, as well as the body sensations that accompany them. Being mindful, or more aware of the things going on in your internal environment, is different than judging or evaluating them.

When you are truly mindful of your thoughts you *notice them without judgment*. It is as if you have stepped outside of your own mind and are looking at your thoughts as an outside observer of them. This allows you to create a safe distance from them and see them as part of who you are without letting them define you. It also allows you to assess how helpful or useful they are without feeling threatened (Hayes, 2005).

When you start to do this, you'll probably notice that a lot of your thoughts and feelings are not very helpful in living a meaningful and productive life. This often happens when your thoughts are really judgments and evaluations instead of observations about the present moment.

As I mentioned in the introduction to this section, internal mindfulness training helps you become more aware of your thoughts, self-talk, mental images, and emotions. One of the key goals of mindfulness training is to learn how to notice and accept your thoughts and feelings instead of spending a lot of time trying to figure out why you are thinking or feeling something, and then trying to avoid, eliminate, or control those thoughts and feelings. The following simple exercise, *What am I Thinking?*, will help you pay more attention to your thinking.

Internal Mindfulness Training Exercise # 1: What Am I Thinking?

Instructions:

1. For the next few minutes write down all of the thoughts that come to mind. Don't analyze them or judge them, just write them down.

____
____
____
____
____
____
____
____
____
____
____
____
____
____
____

2. Label the thoughts with an H, U, S, or B to designate:

   - Helpful—contributes positively to your goals, values, and happiness.
   - Unhelpful—works against your values, and happiness.
   - Silly—absurd silly thoughts.

- Benign—neutral thoughts relative to your goals, values, and happiness

3. Do this activity for a few moments several times a week.
4. At the end of a few weeks, compare your thoughts to the thinking traps discussed earlier.

After a few weeks of noticing your unhelpful thoughts and your thinking traps, you'll be able to identify situations and people that trigger them. You can then use this information to prevent falling into the traps and to manage your unhelpful thinking.

The next level of informal mindfulness training that focuses on your internal environment is paying attention to *the nature of your thoughts*. Besides being helpful or unhelpful, your thoughts can also be examined in terms of whether they are judgments/evaluations or simple observations. Remember, mindfulness is all about noticing, labeling, and accepting. When your mind starts judging and evaluating your thoughts or feelings, it takes you out of the present moment. When this involves sexual thinking it can also lead to sexual response problems. The following exercise, *Sexual Descriptions vs. Judgments* will help you become more aware of the differences between descriptions and judgments.

Internal Mindfulness Training Exercise #2: Sexual Descriptions vs. Judgments

Purpose: As we discussed, informal mindfulness training revolves around increasing attention to the present moment, focusing on the internal and external environments. The purpose of this activity is to help you become more aware of your thoughts about sex and gender without judging or evaluating them.

Instructions:

1. Read each statement and decide whether the statement describes or judges the subject.
2. Put a check mark under either the description or judgment columns.
3. Do not read the answers in the key until you have finished checking off all of the statements.

Statement	**Description**	**Judgment**
1. That woman walking down the beach is wearing a string bikini.		
2. That woman is way too fat to wear any kind of bikini.		
3. That man walking on the beach is wearing a red, white, and blue racing bathing suit.		
4. That man in the racing bathing suit looks ridiculous with his belly hanging out.		
5. He has tan pleated khaki pants on.		
6. Tan pleated khaki pants are so boring.		
7. He has a large bushy mustache.		
8. He needs to trim his moustache.		
9. My first wife was turned on by both men and women.		
10. My first wife was a bisexual. How disgusting.		
11. He likes oral sex a lot.		
12. All he ever thinks about is blow jobs.		

13. She likes me to enter her from the rear when we have intercourse.		
14. She really wants to have anal sex because she likes me to enter her from the rear when we have intercourse.		
15. The average married American couple has intercourse 2-3 times a week.		
16. We don't have sex enough.		
17. We don't have sex as much as we did when we were in our twenties.		
18. Something is wrong with us because we don't have sex as much as we did when we were in our twenties.		
19. It takes me longer to get it up now that I am 60 than it did when I was in my 20s.		
20. I am less of a man because it takes me longer to get it up now that I am 60 than it did when I was in my 20s.		

Go over your answers comparing them to the following key:

Answers:

1.	D	11.	D
2.	J	12.	J
3.	D	13.	D
4.	J	14.	J
5.	D	15.	D
6.	J	16.	J
7.	D	17.	D
8.	J	18.	J
9.	D	19.	D
10.	J	20.	J

Becoming more mindful of your self-talk regarding your sexuality will help you start being more accepting and less judgmental of yourself and others. This pays instant dividends as your partner and significant others begin to feel more appreciated and accepted.

The second area that internal mindfulness training focuses on revolves around what is going on in your body. Using exercises such as the Body Scan to help you become more mindful of generic sensations such as muscle tension throughout your body will help you become more aware of what is going on in your body during your sexual response.

Internal Mindfulness Training
Exercise # 3: Body Scan

Purpose: The following exercise, Body Scan, is designed to help you become more aware of what is going on in your body at any given point in time. It is not intended to help you analyze your body or figure out why your body is the way it is. To do a full Body Scan you'll need about 45 minutes of uninterrupted time and a quiet environment. Try to let go of judgmental and critical thoughts and just follow the script and be aware of the sensations you feel and what is happening in the present moment. There is no right or wrong way to feel while doing this exercise. The way you feel while doing the exercise is the right way to feel. Doing a Body Scan is best performed lying down.

Instructions:
You will find it very helpful to record this script and perform the actions while listening to the recording.

1. Lie on the floor on an exercise or yoga mat. Make sure that your legs are not crossed and your hands are resting comfortably at your sides, palms facing up.
2. Now focus on your breathing.

3. Do not try to change your breathing right now; just notice how the air moves in and out of your body.
4. Notice how your nose feels as air enters your body through it. Focus on this sensation for a couple of breaths.
5. Now notice the feelings and sensations as your breath enters your nose and travels down your windpipe and enters your lungs.
6. Notice how your lungs expand and push against your rib cage.
7. Notice how the muscles attached to your ribs feel as the air enters and leaves your lungs.
8. Focus on the sensations in your ribs for a couple of breaths.
9. Now notice how your abdomen expands gently as your breath enters your body and how your belly moves back in as your breath moves out of your body.
10. Focus on this movement of your belly as you breathe in and out for a couple of breaths.
11. Now imagine that you can see the air enter your nose, go down your windpipe, and fill your lungs as your belly moves in and out with each inhalation and each exhalation. Watch the air fill and empty your lungs for a few breaths.
12. As you breathe in and out comfortably, notice if your mind has wandered.
13. If your mind has wandered from just noticing your breathing, it is ok. Accept the fact that your mind has wandered and shift your attention back to your breathing.
14. Tell yourself *it is ok for my mind to wander. I can accept this without judgment and get back to my breathing.*
15. Now shift your attention to your left foot.
16. Notice the sensations in your left foot and the toes of that foot. Notice the temperature, tension, and anything else you can sense about your foot and toes.
17. Release any tension in your left foot by pointing your toes away from you. Hold this for a few seconds. Now pull the toes of your left foot back towards your head and hold this for a few seconds.

18. Good. Now notice the difference in your left foot after contracting and relaxing it.
19. Repeat this sequence with your right foot.
20. Notice the sensations in your right foot and the toes of that foot. Notice the temperature, tension, and anything else you can sense about your foot and toes.
21. Release any tension in your right foot by pointing your toes away from you. Hold this for a few seconds. Now pull the toes of your right foot back towards your head, and hold this for a few seconds.
22. Good. Now notice the difference in your right foot after contracting and releasing it.
23. Now shift your attention and become aware of the sensations in your lower left leg and knee.
24. Notice the temperature, tension, and anything else you can sense about your lower left leg and knee.
25. Release any tension in your lower left leg and knee by contracting and holding your calf muscle for a few moments. Now bend your left knee and hold it for a few seconds.
26. Good. Now notice the difference in your lower left leg and knee after contracting and releasing it.
27. Now shift your attention and become aware of the sensations in your lower right leg and knee.
28. Notice the temperature, tension, and anything else you can sense about your lower right leg and knee.
29. Release any tension in your lower right leg and knee by contracting and holding your calf muscle for a few moments. Now bend your right knee and hold it for a few seconds.
30. Good. Now notice the difference in your lower right leg and knee after contracting and releasing it.
31. Now shift your attention to the upper part of your left leg, above the knee all the way up to your hip.

32. Notice the temperature, tension, and anything else you can sense about the feelings in the front, sides, and back part of your upper left leg all the way to your hip.
33. Release any tension in your upper left leg by contracting and holding your thigh muscles for a few moments.
34. Good. Now notice the difference in your upper left leg after contracting and releasing it.
35. Now let's shift your attention to the upper part of your right leg, above the knee all the way up to your hip.
36. Notice the temperature, tension, and anything else you can sense about the feelings in the front, sides, and back part of your upper right leg all the way to your hip.
37. Release any tension in your upper right leg by contracting and holding your thigh muscles for a few moments.
38. Good. Now notice the difference in your upper right leg after contracting and releasing it.
39. Now shift your attention to your pelvic area.
40. Notice the sensations in your hips, buttocks, and groin area.
41. Contract this area by tightening your stomach and buttocks. Pull in your stomach and scrunch the muscles in your buttocks. Hold this contraction for a few seconds and then release it.
42. Good. Now notice the difference in your pelvic area after contracting and releasing it.
43. Direct your attention now to your lower back, the region that connects up with your pelvis.
44. Notice the temperature, tension, and anything else you can sense about the feelings in the muscles of your lower back.
45. Contract this area by gently arching your back, keeping your shoulders and buttocks on the floor. Hold this arch for a few seconds and then release it.
46. Good. Now notice the difference in your lower back after contracting and releasing it.
47. Now shift your attention to your upper back.

48. Notice the temperature, tension, and anything else you can sense about the feelings in the muscles of your upper back.
49. Contract this area by gently pulling your shoulders back towards your spine. This will cause your chest to rise and your spine to lift off the floor. Hold this pull for a few seconds and then release it.
50. Good. Now notice the difference in your upper back after contracting and releasing it.
51. Now shift your attention to your left hand and fingers.
52. Notice the temperature, tension, and anything else you can sense about the feelings in the muscles of your left hand and fingers.
53. Contract this area by making a tight fist. Hold this pull for a few seconds and then release it.
54. Good. Now notice the difference in your left hand and fingers after contracting and releasing your fist.
55. Now shift your attention to your right hand and fingers.
56. Notice the temperature, tension, and anything else you can sense about the feelings in the muscles of your right hand and fingers.
57. Contract this area by making a tight fist. Hold this pull for a few seconds and then release it.
58. Good. Now notice the difference in your right hand and fingers after contracting and releasing your fist.
59. Now shift your attention to your lower left arm.
60. Notice the temperature, tension, and anything else you can sense about the feelings in the muscles of your left wrist, forearm, and elbow.
61. You can also contract this area by making a tight fist. Hold this pull for a few seconds and then release it.
62. Good. Now notice the difference in your left wrist, forearm, and elbow after contracting and releasing your fist.
63. Notice the temperature, tension, and anything else you can sense about the feelings in the muscles of your right wrist, forearm, and elbow.

64. You can also contract this area by making a tight fist. Hold this pull for a few seconds and then release it.
65. Good. Now notice the difference in your left wrist, forearm, and elbow after contracting and releasing your fist.
66. Now shift your attention to your upper left arm all the way to your armpit.
67. Notice the temperature, tension, and anything else you can sense about the feelings in the muscles of your upper left arm all the way to your armpit.
68. Contract this area by making a tight fist and curling it up to your shoulder. Hold this pull for a few seconds and then release it.
69. Good. Now notice the difference in your upper left arm after contracting and releasing your fist .
70. Now shift your attention to your upper right arm all the way to your armpit.
71. Notice the temperature, tension, and anything else you can sense about the feelings in the muscles of your upper right arm all the way to your armpit.
72. Contract this area by making a tight fist and curling it up to your shoulder. Hold this pull for a few seconds and then release it.
73. Good. Now notice the difference in your upper right arm after contracting and releasing your fist.
74. Now shift your attention to your shoulders.
75. Notice the temperature, tension, and anything else you can sense about the feelings in the muscles of your shoulders.
76. Contract this area by shrugging your shoulders up towards your ears. Try to touch your ears with your shoulders. Hold this shrug for a few seconds and then release it.
77. Good. Now notice the difference in your shoulders after contracting and releasing your fist.
78. Now shift your attention to your neck and the base of your skull.

79. Notice the temperature, tension, and anything else you can sense about the feelings in the muscles of your neck and the base of your skull.
80. Contract this area by gently pulling your chin towards your chest. Keep your shoulders on the floor while doing this. Hold this shrug for a few seconds and then release it.
81. Good. Now notice the difference in your neck and the base of your skull after contracting and releasing your fist.
82. Now shift your attention to your face.
83. Notice the temperature, tension, and anything else you can sense about the feelings in the muscles of your lips, mouth, chin, and jaw.
84. Contract this area by scrunching your chin, cheek, and forehead by making the silliest face possible. Hold this silly face for a few seconds and then release it.
85. Good. Now notice the difference in your face after contracting and releasing it.
86. Now shift your attention to your entire body.
87. Notice the sensations in your body as you relax and refocus on the present moment.
88. Slowly wiggle your toes and fingers, stretch and flex your arms and hands, and take a few deep breaths.
89. When you are ready you may sit up or stand and get ready to resume your daily activities, refreshed and calm.

Regular practice of this form of mindfulness will help you become more aware of what is going on in your body during sexual activities of any kind. It will help you learn to sharpen your focus and keep your mind from drifting when you make love with your partner.

Focus on the External Environment

As I discussed previously, your external environment includes your behavior and your physical environment. Behavior is a catchall term for all of your actions, whether intentional or unintentional. Your environment includes everything in your immediate personal surroundings from the interior of your car to the sensual environment of your bedroom. Unlike your thoughts and feelings, which come and go on their own and are beyond your conscious control, you can control your behavior and your personal environment. You can decide how to act and how to manage your personal sexual environment. These can greatly impact your personal sexuality and your sexual relationships.

External Mindfulness Exercise # 1: Letting Go

Purpose: Paying attention to the present moment involves catching your mind when it shifts focus to the past or the future, and then redirecting your full attention back to your behavior, what you're doing now. The following non-sexual exercise, *Letting Go,* is designed to help you do this by focusing on common items in your external environment. This exercise revolves around becoming more mindful of how you touch and then let go of things. It is a simple but effective way to remind you to slow down and pay attention to what you are doing in the present moment.

Instructions:

1. For the next 24 hours pay attention every time your hand lets go of something. This could involve letting go of a cup or glass, door handle, cabinet or drawer pull, your pen, or another person's hand.
2. Be mindful of exactly what's going on and write down the details of how you let things go and the consequences of your actions.
3. Note how you put that glass down. Notice the movement of the doorknob when you turn it slowly and gently close the door or when you forget and just release it from your fingers.

4. Pay attention to the texture, weight, shape, and feel of everything you handle and let go of.
5. Note how paying attention to these things influences how you release them.
6. Describe the consequences of the way you let go of things today. Did you get a certain look from a person when you released his or her hand? Did a door or drawer slam (or not slam) when you were mindful of how you released it?
7. When the day is over, write down what you've learned from this activity.
8. If you practiced this on a regular basis, how do you think being more mindful of letting go could impact your life and slow you down?

(Anderson Krech, 1966, Krech, 2005).

Another great nonsexual exercise for becoming more mindful of the external environment focuses on visual sensations. We often miss out on details in our immediate environment because we do not pay attention to the world around us. We walk around with our mind racing into the future and our eyes focused on our phones or just staring blindly ahead without really seeing. External mindfulness training activity revolves around increasing your attention to the present moment and your immediate environment.

External Mindfulness Training Exercise # 2: Eight Shades of .....

Purpose: The purpose of the next exercise, entitled *Eight Shades of* ….. is to help you stop, observe, and be aware of common things in your immediate environment without judging or evaluating them.

Instructions:

1. Choose a color to observe.
2. Go for a walk at lunchtime and find 8 tints or shades of this color in items in or around your home or work environment.
3. Describe the objects you selected that had your color.
4. Describe how the color varied across the different objects you chose.
5. Write down one thing you learned from this exercise about mindfulness (Krech, 2005).

Another way to increase your external mindfulness is to practice mindful eating. Mindful eating activities focus on two dimensions of the external environment—your personal eating behavior and the context in which it occurs (your immediate physical environment). In other words, they look at how you eat and the circumstances surrounding your eating.

Mindful eating is often taught to people with eating disorders to help them become more mindful of their eating behavior. Some of the variables involved in this include:

- Setting the table and paying attention to the aesthetics of the eating environment.
- Sitting quietly and observing the food before eating it.
- Cutting food into small pieces.
- Slowly picking up the pieces and lifting the food off the plates and bringing it to their mouths.
- Taking slow bites and chewing thoroughly.

Eating this way helps people experience their food like never before. They begin to marvel at things like how the fingers, hands, and arms work in consort with their brain to pick the food up and bring it into the mouth, the process of chewing, the experience of tasting something anew.

The purpose of this book does not revolve around using mindful eating to treat eating disorders. I've used the next two exercises in my sex coaching practice because they are also excellent sensuality training activities.

External Mindfulness Training Exercise #3: The Sensuous Orange

Purpose: This activity is designed to help you become more mindful of your external environment and become more sensuous by focusing all five of your senses while peeling and eating an orange. The exercise has two parts.

Instructions

Part 1: Shopping

1. Buy a navel orange. Choose an orange that is easy to peel.
2. Try to find one that is not "perfect" (perfectly round and perfectly orange).
3. Look for an orange that has a distinctive color, with imperfections.

Part 2: Peeling and Eating

1. With your eyes closed, do the following things:

    - Pick up the orange and feel its weight.
    - Feel the shape of the orange.
    - Roll the orange around your face and neck and feel the temperature of the orange.
    - Put it up to your nose and smell it.
    - Roll it over your ears and hear it.

2. Now open your eyes and do the following things:

    - Notice the size and shape of the orange.
    - Notice the color of the orange.
    - Notice the texture of the orange.
    - Notice any distinguishing characteristics of the orange (bruises, imperfections, etc.).

3. Now I want you to peel the orange by keeping it in one piece:

    - Make a small incision at the top of the orange with your fingernail or a knife.
    - Slowly peel the orange from the top to the bottom.
    - Notice the peeling process and what is going on in your mind and the orange as you peel it.
    - Break off a piece of the peel and twist it to get the oil.
    - Feel, smell, and taste the orange oil.

4. Now I want you to take one section of the orange and do the following:

    - Notice how the orange section is constructed.
    - Peel back a small section of the casing, the cellulose wrapper that keeps it together.
    - Take out one individual orange sperm.
    - Close your eyes, put it on your tongue, and pop it with your tongue.

5. Now I want you to close your eyes and eat the one section of the orange this way:

    - Nibble the orange section, don't gulp it.
    - Slowly chew each small bite.
    - Slowly swallow each small bite.
    - Notice your thoughts and feelings as you eat the orange section.

6. Finish eating the orange.
7. Answer the following questions:

   - How did your thoughts about eating an orange differ from actually eating it?
   - What did you notice about the orange? Peeling it? Eating it?
   - What new thing did you learn about oranges?

The next exercise also involves mindful eating and takes the experience to the next sexual level by doing it in bed and using it as a prelude to more erotic activities with your partner.

External Mindfulness Training
Exercise # 4: Mindful Eating and Drinking in Bed

Purpose: The purpose of this activity is to help you become more mindful by stopping, observing, and being aware of one concrete activity you engage in daily: eating. Combining this with the location (on your bed) also makes it a sensuality-building activity. This is a two-part activity. Part one involves shopping. Part two involves mindful eating in bed.

Instructions Part 1:

1. Purchase the following items: a naval orange, a pear, an apple, a bunch of red and green grapes, two boxes of different crackers, two different types of cheeses, a bottle of red or white wine.
2. Prepare the fruit, cheese, and crackers by sectioning the fruit, cutting pieces of the cheese, and putting some crackers on a big tray.
3. Pour two glasses of wine and bring them and the rest of the bottle to the bedside.

Instructions Part 2:

1. Choose a piece of fruit and eat it as you normally would. (Have your partner also do this.)

2. Now choose another piece of fruit and do the following instead of just quickly eating it:

    - Notice the size, shape, and color of the piece of fruit.
    - Feel the texture, weight, and temperature of the piece.
    - Now close your eyes, slowly bring the piece of fruit to your nose, and smell it.
    - Notice the aromas emanating from the fruit.

3. Now slowly bring the item to your ear and listen to it.
4. Notice any sounds it makes as you hold it to your ear.
5. With your eyes still closed, put the piece in your mouth and let it rest on your tongue for a while.
6. After a few moments chew the item slowly.
7. Chew it at least ten times before swallowing it.
8. Repeat step two with each different item on your tray.
9. In between sampling the different items on your tray, stop, take a sip of wine, and do the following:

    - Notice the size, shape, and color of your wine glass with the wine in it.
    - Feel the texture, weight, and temperature of the glass as you hold it in your hand.
    - Now close your eyes, slowly bring the glass to your nose, and smell it.
    - Notice the aromas emanating from the wine.
    - With your eyes still closed, take a sip of the wine and swirl it around your mouth but do not swallow it.
    - Notice the taste, texture, and temperature of the wine.

10. Now swallow the wine and notice how it feels as it slides down your throat and reaches your stomach.
11. Continue to sip and experience the wine as you eat your fruit, cheese, and crackers.

12. Take turns feeding yourself and your partner.

Have your partner close their eyes as you feed them individual pieces of fruit, cheese, and crackers.

13. Take your time and finish the food and drink at your own pace. You may use this as a prelude to making love or just as a fun snack time in bed.
14. Write down your thoughts, self-talk, mental images, and emotions related to thinking about and then doing this activity.

You can change the foods chosen for this exercise to suit your food preferences and allergies. There are many different food and wine combinations. Pick one that works for you. Instead of peeling an orange you might want to use a tangerine. If you are not a wine or alcohol drinker you can substitute seltzer or another non-alcoholic choice.

Part 3
Sexual Mindfulness

Introduction to Part Three

In section three you'll combine your knowledge of the components of sexuality with the actual practice of mindfulness. I'll show you how to use techniques from Acceptance and Commitment Therapy and Japanese Psychology to work with your mind instead of against it as it creates helpful and unhelpful thoughts, self-talk, mental images, and emotions related to sex. I call this unleashing your sexual mind.

The whole idea of part three is to use your mindfulness training to shift the focus off of yourself and your troubling thoughts and painful emotions and onto your partner for the good of the relationship. I'm assuming at this point that one of the reasons you bought this book and got this far in reading it is that you place a high value on your relationship and the sexual aspects of it.

This is important because, whenever you get stuck on some of the exercises or content in section three, I want you to think about it as behaving in a way that serves your sexual relationship and is consistent with your values. Say to yourself: "In the service of strengthening my sexual relationship with my partner, I am willing to accept the troubling thoughts and painful emotions that this exercise/content is triggering."

Looking at the new exercise or material from this perspective will help you co-exist with your troubling thoughts and painful feelings as you try something new and challenging because you value your sexual relationship more than being in your outdated comfort zone.

You'll notice that in the last five chapters there are several erotic and explicitly sexual exercises. Some of them are bound to upset you in some way. As you read through the exercises you'll notice the following dialogue:

> *Notice your thoughts, self-talk, mental images, and feelings, as you massage your partner's back. If your mind wanders into the future or the past or fills with unhelpful thoughts and feelings note that this is happening*

and say to yourself, "There goes my runaway mind again, taking me out of the present moment," and refocus on your attention on your partner's body and the sensations in your hands and fingers as you massage.

This example is taken from the back massage exercise in chapter 14. I repeat these mindful self-reflection instructions throughout the exercises in chapters 14 (massage) 15 (masturbation), 16 (oral sex) and 17 (sexual intercourse). I understand that for some readers some of the content in these chapters might be very upsetting and will challenge some of your religious or moral teachings. I urge you to read the material anyway and try to view it from the perspective of using it to provide pleasure to your partner for the good of the relationship. Maintaining the passion in long-term sexual relationships is not always easy, especially if you and your partner have different levels of sexual desire and interest or different religious/moral/ethical values. Once again I urge you to be mindful of those values and the thoughts and feelings they trigger and discuss this with your partner.

Try to think about doing sexual favors for your partner the same way you would think of doing other favors for him/her. You see movies, travel to certain places, visit relatives, eat in certain restaurants, do household chores, spend money, and do a hundred other things for your partner that you probably would not do if he/she didn't ask you to. Why not start to look at sexual favors the same way, as things you do in the service of the relationship? Think of it as a special category of giving that you share with grace and gratitude. This isn't a blanket acceptance of anything your partner desires. If something really goes against your morals, ethics, or values you should discuss this. Obviously if your partner wants you to do something physically harmful or illegal you have the right to refuse.

Chapter 11

Clarifying Your Sexual Values

Your values are the mirror of your personality and are central to defining who you are as a sexual person. Your values serve as the roadmap for your life and the direction it takes. They reflect your morals and ethics and are the foundation of your personality. You have values related to a number of things, including sex. Your sexual values cover all six aspects of your sexual identity—your biological sex, gender identity, gender role, sexual orientation, sexual behavior, and sexual response. One of the primary goals for practicing sexual mindfulness is behaving in ways that are consistent (congruent) with your sexual values. This is called values-congruent behavior. Understanding your sexual values will also help you set values-congruent sexual goals for yourself and your relationship.

Most people view values as fixed and immutable. In fact, your values are fluid and can change as you age and are exposed to new information and experiences. Some of your values won't change completely, they just bend a little, as trees do when confronted by the winds. Think of each of the components of your sexual identity as branches of your values tree. Your values tree has deep roots that nurture and sustain your sexual values. When a tree is confronted by heavy winds, it has the ability to bend without its branches breaking. When your values tree is confronted by the winds of change in your life, the more psychological flexibility you have, the more likely your branches (your sexual values) will be to bend without breaking from the strain.

Unfortunately, most people are not psychologically flexible enough to accept this. Instead of viewing values as fluid and capable of change, they view them as fixed and unchangeable. They feel threatened by the idea that their values can change and try to control, avoid, or eliminate the troubling thoughts and painful emotions aroused by this. They resist accepting their changing values because they conflict with the values they were raised with. A more psychologically flexible person sees their changing values as a healthy adaptation to the growth that accompanies exposure to new information, ideas, and experiences.

Improving your sexual relationship with your partner can be greatly enhanced by understanding your sexual values and how they mesh or clash with your partner. Since your sexual values are central to who you are as a person and what gives your life meaning and purpose, living in sync with them is a great source of happiness. Being in a relationship with someone who has very different sexual values can be a tremendous source of stress and a great strain on the partnership.

Let me give you an example. Ted, a senior in one of my Human Sexuality classes, came to talk to me about Laura, a new partner he had been dating for a couple of months. He told me that he loved everything about her. She was attractive, intelligent, witty, athletic, and shared his passion for the great outdoors. He had been spending a lot of time with her and told me, "She could be the one. She could be the one person I'd really consider committing myself to." The only problem, he said, was that Laura had different sexual values than he did. I asked him what he meant and he explained that she valued the physical aspect of sex much more than he did. While he enjoyed kissing and cuddling and *making love* with her, she just wanted to *fuck* more than make love. The sheer intensity of her lust scared him. Sometimes, he said, it seemed that he was only an object that she used to satisfy her sexual needs. He worried about being able to keep up with Laura and satisfy her sexually. While he enjoyed kissing, cuddling, making love, and having an orgasm, this seemed like just a warm-up for her. He explained that she liked to spend the whole morning (or afternoon, or evening) in bed having sex. He preferred to do something else after making love. He didn't want to spend hours in bed. He really wasn't sure what to do about their differences. He loved everything about her and wanted to please her, but sex just wasn't as important to him as it was to her. He simply didn't value it as much as Laura did. He felt stuck and did not know how to proceed. He and

Laura were graduating in three months and had started talking about moving in together after college ended.

I lost track of Ted after that and about two years later he dropped by my office. He was working in the area and stopped by during his lunch break. He told me that he and Laura had recently gotten married and they were doing ok. I asked him how the sex was going, and he said that things were great. They had reached a natural point in their relationship and it seemed to be working out. He told me that Laura still had a higher sex drive than him, but ever since they moved in together and could have sex whenever they wanted she seemed to be content to not want to spend entire mornings or afternoons in bed. In fact, they were having sex more often, but not spending as much time actually having sex. He said that since they were working full-time and living together it had just worked out that way.

Core and Satellite Values

There are two different levels of values: core and satellite values. Each plays a role in understanding your sexual values. Your core values represent the things that are central to who you are and are non-negotiable. Your core values are the bedrock of your personality and include things like your country, spouse, children, religion, and freedom. Your satellite values consist of less important things that you hold dear but aren't as strongly committed to. Satellite values typically include political beliefs, cultural traditions, community service, personal attributes (intelligence, beauty, and so on), hobbies, recreational activities, sports, and so forth.

You have core and satellite values related to your sexuality and sexual relationships. There are things about your sexual relationship that you consider nonnegotiable and are central to your happiness (core values), while other aspects are much less important (satellite values) and are negotiable. There are many ways to assess your core and satellite values. There are four steps involved in clarifying your values:

1. Exploring values
2. Choosing and ranking values
3. Publicly affirming values
4. Acting on values

The rest of this chapter is devoted to using exercises to explore each of these steps. The first exercise that I use with my students and clients is called "A Perfect Day." It uses everyday activities to reflect your underlying values. It is also a good first look at how much you value sex in general. This exercise is modified from one developed by Krech, 2005.

Values Exercise # 1 (Exploring): A Perfect Day

Purpose: Think about the perfect day that reflects all of your values. If you could plan a perfect day, what specific things would you do? Who would be with you when you did these things? Where would you do these things? Would your activities include work, play, community service? I want you to think of these activities as your Daily Life Criteria (DLC) for a perfect day. Your DLCs must be concrete activities. Instead of saying something like "relaxing," say "lying by a pool with my partner" or "meditating under a tree." Other than that, let your imagination go wild and not be restricted by place and time.

Instructions:

1. List up to ten daily life criteria for a perfect day:

____

____

____

____

____

____

____

2. How do your DLCs reflect your core and satellite values?
3. How your DLCs compare to those of your partner?
4. How big of a part does sex play in your perfect day?
5. How does your typical day compare to your perfect day?
6. What stands in your way of meeting your DLCs for a perfect day?
7. Describe a specific way that you could incorporate one of your DLCs into a typical day regardless of the things standing in your way.

The more you live in sync with your daily life criteria, the more your life will be driven by your own values, not those of others. Another really powerful tool to help you assess your values and put things into perspective is to look at your life and use of time. This is particularly powerful if you have reached midlife and realize that half of your time on the planet is already over.

The following exercise, "Thirty Thousand Days," helps you do just that. It is based on the average life span for Americans of 80 years (roughly 30,00 days). While some people live much longer than this and some die much younger, it provides a good baseline for looking at how you want to spend the rest of your life. This exercise is modified from one developed by Krech, 2005.

Values Exercise #2 (Exploring): Thirty Thousand Days

Purpose: The exercise is designed to help you assess your values by having you look at the remaining time you have left on the planet and how you want to use it. I've found that this activity has more meaning the older one is. The first time I did it, I was blown away by how powerful it was. I'd lived more than half of my life and realized that there were still things I was doing that I didn't want to do. I also realized that I was spending time with people who brought me down and didn't contribute to my life's purpose. I've found that students and clients in their forties and fifties react the same way. Sometimes younger people aren't as moved by its power.

Instructions:

1. Count the number of full years you've lived up until this year and multiply those by 365.
2. Next, add up all the days (including today) that you've lived this year.
3. Add these numbers together to calculate the exact number of days you've lived so far.
4. Subtract this number from 30,000. This is the approximate number of days you have left on earth.
5. Make up the following three lists: (a) Things I want to start doing, (b) Things I want to continue doing, and (c) Things I want to stop doing.
6. Describe how you want to spend the rest of your life using information gathered from these three lists.
7. How does sex factor into your three lists?

When you do this exercise it helps you focus on the things in your life that matter the most. The things on your lists represent your values and their importance is emphasized by their relationship to the time left to explore them. This exercise helps you examine where you put sex on your priority list. It also sets the stage for accepting this and co-existing with it as you work with your partner to strengthen your relationship.

Values Exercise # 3 (Exploring): Sorting the Mail

Purpose: Exploring sexual values can get pretty confusing. One useful way to do this is to sort through them like sorting through the mail. You put each value in a separate "mail slot" (aka manila envelope) that matches a sexual value category.

Instructions:

1. Get five manila folders or large envelopes and label them with the following category titles:

    - Gender Identity Values
    - Gender Role Values
    - Sexual Orientation Values
    - Sexual Behavior Values
    - Sexual Relationship Values

2. On 5" x 8" file cards, answer the following values questions for each category:

    - What exactly do I value about this category?

Example: What exactly do I value about sexual relationships?
I value having someone who shares my love.
I value the physical contact I get with another human being.
I value having a single steady sexual partner.
I value having someone with whom I can share my deepest thoughts and feelings.
I value having a close companion to share things with.

3. Take your time as you work through each values category.
4. Do not judge your values; just accept them for what they are and put them in their proper place. You'll rank them later. For now, just spend the time categorizing and sorting them.

Choosing and ranking values is the next step in defining valued directions. Ranking values will help you distinguish your core values from your satellite ones. This allows you to identify areas of negotiation and compromise, two things that are essential to healthy sexual relationships. As we discussed, your core sexual values represent the things that you are not willing to change and are nonnegotiable, while your satellite sexual values consist of less important things that are negotiable. If you know your core and satellite sexual values, and those of your partner, it will give you a greater understanding of how your thoughts and feelings about this relate to getting stuck.

Values Exercise # 4: Choosing and Ranking Your Values

Purpose: This activity builds on the previous one in this chapter by helping you rank your sexual values.

Instructions:

1. Look at the five folders/envelopes you set up in the previous exercise.
2. Rank each folder/envelope in order of its importance (1 = the highest).
3. On a table or the floor put the most important envelope in the middle and arrange the remaining four around it.
4. Take all of the sexual values cards out of the envelopes and put them into five piles, keeping the most important pile in the middle with the other piles surrounding it.
5. Starting with the pile in the middle, read each value a few times.
6. Use numbers to rank each of the values contained in this pile from most important to least important.
7. Line up all of these cards in order of their importance.
8. Step back three feet from these cards and tell yourself:

"These are my most deeply held sexual values."

"I accept them for what they are."

"I realize that some of them may not be helpful in meeting my current sexual goals and can be replaced."

9. Repeat step 8 for each of the piles.
10. Go back to the piles and see if there are any values you feel differently about now that you have identified and ranked them.
11. Discard any of the outdated and unhelpful values or replace them with new, more helpful ones.

One final exercise, Clarifying Your Values, combines all four elements of the Defining Valued Directions process in a very simple but powerful way.

Values Exercise # 5: Clarifying Your Values

Purpose: This activity combines all four elements of the Defining Valued Directions processes. It will help you clarify your sexual values and set the stage for writing values-based sexual relationship goals.

Instructions:

1. Explore what you value. Pick one of your core sexual values from the pile of values you put in the middle of the circle. Copy what you wrote on that card on these lines:

____

____

2. Rank this value. Write down the rank you gave this value from the "Core vs. Satellite Values" exercise:

____

____

3. Publicly affirm. Some things I can do to affirm this value to others are:

____

____

4. Take action. Some things I can do to demonstrate this value to others are:

____

____

5. Identify the things that make it difficult to affirm and act on your values. The thoughts, self-talk, scary pictures, or emotions that make it difficult for me to speak about this value or act on it are:

____

6. Identify what you are willing to accept. I'm willing to accept the following to affirm and act on this value:

____

____

Example:

1. Explore what you value. "Having sex with my partner at least 3-4 times/week."
2. Rank this value. "I ranked this #1."
3. Publicly affirm. "I could talk in private to my partner about it."
4. Take action. "I can write a note to my partner expressing my desire to have sex with her more often."
5. Identify the things that make it difficult to affirm and act on your values. "I am afraid to upset my partner by telling her I want sex this often. I don't want to come off as demanding and am afraid she will reject me. I close my eyes and see her getting mad and walking out of the room on me."

6. Identify what you are willing to accept. "I'm willing to accept the risk of upsetting her and having her walk out. I am willing to accept my fear and anxiety related to this."
7. You are going to use information from this activity to set new sexual and relationship goals.
8. By setting goals that are consistent with what you value, it will increase the likelihood of attaining them.

When you have completed these exercises, you are ready to use this information to set new values-congruent sexual and relationship goals. By setting goals that are consistent with what you value, it will increase the likelihood of attaining them.

CHAPTER 12

Sexual Acceptance and Commitment

Sexual acceptance and commitment training build upon your mindfulness skills and values work. Now that you are more aware of what your sexual values are, you need to figure out what you are going to do with that information to enhance your relationship. Acceptance and commitment training will help you figure this out. Acceptance has four components:

- Accepting reality for what it is
- Accepting what you can and cannot control
- Accepting that trying to avoid, eliminate, or control troubling thoughts and painful emotions actually makes them worse
- Accepting that the best way to manage troubling thoughts and painful emotions is to accept them and co-exist with them, as you shift your focus off of them and onto taking values-congruent action (Blonna, 2010)

All four of these components can be applied to sexuality-related issues.

Accepting Reality For What it Is

The Japanese call this *arugamama*, accepting reality for what it is. Accepting reality for what it is implies two things: (1) you accept whatever troubling thoughts and painful feelings you are experiencing at the moment, and (2) you accept that experiencing troubling thoughts and painful feelings is part of being human (Morita, 1998).

If you can accept reality for what it is you can begin to shift your attention away from your troubling thoughts and painful emotions and onto something productive. In time, the negative thoughts and emotions fade as your focus is directed away from them.

Accepting something and being willing to move forward while coexisting with it doesn't mean you necessarily want it. It just means that you admit that it exists and you don't deny it. It also means that you accept the fact that most of the worthwhile goals you set for yourself will not come easy and will involve sacrifice, discipline, pain, and suffering, as well as the troubling thoughts and painful emotions that go with them. You accept the reality of your pain and suffering as a starting point for dealing with it.

Accepting What You Can and Cannot Control

Acceptance training helps you learn how to accept things that are beyond your control. As we discussed in chapter two of this book, there are two sets of factors related to control: internal factors and external factors. Internal factors are the things that go on in your mind— your thoughts, self-talk, mental images, and emotions. These internal factors come and go like the wind and most are beyond your conscious control. For example, if I told you to "feel happy," you could not simply close your eyes and conjure up happiness. Similarly, you could not summon up sadness, lust, or any other feeling.

External factors relate to your behavior and your environment. While you cannot control most of your thoughts or feelings, you can control your behavior. This is especially true in relationships. You can choose how you behave in relation to your thoughts and feelings. There is a relationship between behavior and thoughts and feelings (Hayes, 2005).

For instance, you can trigger happy feelings by doing something that you know makes you feel joy. For example, I know from past experience that giving my wife a back or foot rub triggers feelings of love and tenderness in me. If I want to experience those emotions, I can't just will myself to feel them. I can, however, trigger them by doing something—giving her a back or foot rub.

You also have some degree of control over your microenvironment (living room, bedroom, etc.). You can make modifications to any of these to enhance your sexuality and relationship (sensual sheets, candles, good music, etc.).

Accepting That Trying to Avoid, Eliminate, or Control Troubling Thoughts and Painful Emotions Actually Makes Them Worse

The most important aspect of acceptance is the fact that when you try to avoid, control, or eliminate troubling thoughts and painful feelings, *they actually worsen.* Research shows that focusing your attention and self-talk on trying to avoid, control, or eliminate painful thoughts and feelings actually *increases your suffering* (Hayes et al, 1999).

In his book *Get Out of Your Mind and into Your Life*, Steve Hayes (2005) points out that acceptance isn't easy. Accepting the troubling thoughts and self-talk, scary pictures, and painful emotions that at times flood your mind can seem overwhelming. In many cases, you've carried them around for years, and it's been very difficult to get rid of them. You've probably spent a lot of time trying to avoid, control or eliminate them in the past. The problem with doing this is that it actually increases your focus on them and keeps them in the forefront of your consciousness. This keeps them alive rather than letting them dissipate on their own.

Accepting something doesn't mean you necessarily *want* it. It just means that you admit that it exists and you don't deny it. You accept the existence of your troubling thoughts and painful feelings as a starting point for dealing with what triggered them.

For example, you might not like the anger you feel toward your spouse this morning about something she said to you, but you accept that it exists and are willing to help her get the kids ready for school. You accept the fact that you can be angry at something she said or did, and still respect and love her and be willing to work with her.

This shows that you can be psychologically flexible and manage these seemingly contradictory positions.

You don't really want to feel angry at your wife (or anyone for that matter), and you don't necessarily like the sensations that anger creates in your body. You realize that you'd prefer to feel something other than anger, but you accept it and are willing to move forward despite it.

Accepting that the best way to manage painful internal factors is to accept them and co-exist with them, as you shift your focus off of them and onto taking values-congruent action.

Instead of trying to control, avoid, or eliminate your troubling thoughts and painful emotions, the best way to deal with them is to accept them and co-exist with them. In the previous example, that involved focusing on helping your wife get the kids ready for school.

A key component of coexisting with troubling thoughts and painful emotions while taking valued action is learning how to shift your focus off of them and onto behavior that is congruent with your values. Instead of ruminating about what your wife said, you focus on doing what needs to be done to get the kids off to school. Making this kind of mental shift will eventually take your mind off of yourself and your problems.

ACT uses a lot of metaphors to help people understand concepts like control. A fun metaphor I developed to help you visualize the issue of control is called the Mp3 Player.

Acceptance and Commitment Exercise # 1: The Mp3 Player

Purpose: A simple way to help you understand the relationship between willingness and control is to think of them as the metaphor exemplified by an Mp3 Player. This metaphor shows how control and willingness to take values-congruent action are inversely related. It uses the visual representation of up and down volume keys on an Mp3 player to represent the relationship between willingness and control.

Instructions:

1. Read the following metaphor:

Imagine you are going out for a run. You are all ready to go, so you put your portable Mp3 player in your arm holder, insert your ear buds and are ready to rock and roll. The player is compact, has ear bud speakers, selection and volume controls, and a button with an up-and-down arrow to regulate the bass and treble functions. When you want to increase the treble, you press and hold the up arrow, and the treble increases When you want to increase the bass, you press and hold the down arrow, and the bass increases.

These functions work in opposition of each other. As you increase the treble, the bass decreases, and vice versa. Now imagine that instead of regulating the treble and bass, the up-and-down arrow regulates acceptance and control. The next time you have troubling thoughts and painful emotions related to sex that you're trying to control, imagine that you're hooked up to your Mp3 player and have your thumb on the up-and-down arrow.

Press and hold the down arrow (the control function) and notice how you increase your desire to control your thoughts, self-talk, mental images and emotions. As you continue to press and hold the control arrow, you are less and less accepting and willing to take action.

Now press and hold the up arrow (the acceptance function) and notice how this begins to reverse. As your acceptance increases you become more and more willing to take action while coexisting with your troubling thoughts and painful emotions. Notice how your need to control decreases as your acceptance and willingness to take action increases.

Whenever you get stuck and realize you're trying to control your troubling thoughts and painful emotions, close your eyes and imagine the Mp3 Player. Visualize putting your finger on the willingness arrow, and feel your desire to control start to fade. You might want to say to yourself, *I'm having those old urges to control things again. It is time to get out my Mp3 Player and go for a run.* This simple exercise will help you regain your focus and trigger a natural reduction of your troubling thoughts and painful emotions.

The Serenity Prayer

Hayes (1984) has used the Serenity Prayer to illustrate the connection between acceptance and commitment and spirituality. I remember the Serenity Prayer, carved into a wood plaque, sitting above my third-grade classroom chalkboard in public school in Newark, New Jersey: "God grant me the serenity to accept the things I cannot change, the courage to change those that I can, and the wisdom to know the difference."

In a sense, this little prayer captures the essence of acceptance and commitment. ACT clearly supports the first two components of the prayer. Acceptance of things you cannot change—like your past, and your thoughts, personal scripts, scary pictures, and painful emotions—is central to ACT. Being willing to take valued action—while coexisting with your stressful thoughts, scripts, scary pictures, and painful emotions—takes courage. ACT acknowledges this and helps you accept the pain and suffering inherent in your life while helping you find the courage to take valued action.

Where ACT differs from religious interpretations of the prayer is where the "wisdom to know the difference" comes in. The religious interpretation believes that God or some supernatural power provides the wisdom. In essence, a religious interpretation implies that if you follow the teachings of your religion, it'll provide the wisdom you need to know the difference. Using an ACT interpretation, the wisdom to know the difference doesn't come from the supernatural; it comes from contextual and behavioral science which have provided the wisdom to know that the difference involves your behavior and your environment (Hayes 2001, 2004b). You have the wisdom to know the difference between what you can and cannot change in your life. You can change your behavior and your environment despite the events of the past and the intellectual and emotional baggage that you carry around inside your head every day. You don't have to be a slave to your past that keeps you stuck and limits your psychological flexibility.

A useful exercise to help you learn how to accept your troubling thoughts and painful feelings while committing to take action is called *A Six Step-Action Plan for Coexisting With Your Painful Feelings.*

Acceptance and Commitment Exercise # 2: A Six-Step Action Plan for Coexisting With Your Painful Feelings

Purpose: Most people want to avoid troubling thoughts and painful feelings. They avoid potential stressors that trigger them. The following exercise, *Six-Step Action Plan for Coexisting With Your Feelings,* is designed to teach you a simple technique for recognizing, accepting, and coexisting with troubling thoughts and painful emotions.

Instructions:

1. This week, pay closer attention to your painful emotions related to your sexual relationship.
2. Don't question them or try to figure out *why* you are feeling them. Merely note what you are feeling.
3. When you get stuck trying to avoid, control, or eliminate your painful sexual emotions, use the following six steps to help you manage them:

Step 1. Identify the feeling. Pay close attention to exactly how the emotion feels and make note of it in the following nonjudgmental manner, using anxiety as the example:

Isn't this interesting. I am pissed off at my husband again after something he said about last night's lovemaking. I notice that whenever I get angry by something he does, my neck muscles start to tighten, my hands get clammy, and I start to breathe more rapidly and in a shallow fashion.

Step 2. Accept the feeling. Tell yourself:

I am definitely feeling angry. I'd rather not feel this way but I guess it is normal to feel like this when you fight with your husband the first thing in the morning when you have to get the kids ready to go to school.

Step 3. Tell yourself that you can co-exist with these feelings and still take action. Here is an example:

I would prefer not to get angry so easily. I don't really like feeling this way, but I can handle it.

Step 4. Redirect Your Focus. Rather than focus on your emotions, redirect your focus to something that needs to be done. For instance, in this example you could focus completely on making the kids' lunches. Give each lunch your undivided attention and when your thoughts drift back to your husband, redirect them to your lunch preparations.

Step 5. Get physical. If possible, try to do something physical as soon as your thoughts and feelings get the best of you. Maybe you could walk the kids to the school bus stop and then continue walking for a while after they get picked up.

Step 6. Reinforce your ability to co-exist. Remind yourself that you can co-exist with your anger while doing what needs to be done to take care of your kids and yourself.

In time, accepting your troubling thoughts and painful feelings and co-existing with them will become part of your daily routine. This will show you that you do not have to be a slave to troubling thoughts and painful feelings. You can co-exist with them and take productive action despite them.

Sexual Commitment

Commitment is the action component of acceptance. Acceptance is something that goes on in your mind while commitment involves acting on your values-based goals. Now that you are more mindful of your sexual values and accept them, it is time to take action.

As we discussed, a big part of sexual mindfulness is taking values-congruent action in order to have the kind of sexual relationship you want and deserve. This involves setting clear sexual goals and committing to seeing them through while co-existing with the troubling thoughts and painful emotions that will often accompany them.

Setting Values-Based Sexual Goals and Objectives

Goals and objectives go hand-in-hand. Think of your *goals* as having your head in the clouds, while your *objectives* are having your feet planted firmly on the ground. Having your head in the clouds allows you to dream about the kind of sex life you really want. Having your feet on the ground gives you a workable game plan for how to get there and measure your success. Effective goals are ones that are based on are measurable objectives. Any goals that are not based on measurable objectives are unrealistic and much more likely to be unmet.

Goals are broad statements that are not necessarily measurable, such as: *I want to have a great sex life with my partner, I want to have a happy marriage,* or *I want to have a more adventurous sex life.* Measurable objectives are action-oriented. They are based on behavioral outcomes that can be quantified. Objectives are tightly written statements that answer the question, *Who, will do how much, of what, by when?* Examples of objectives are: *By the end of next month I will try out two new intercourse positions with my partner; for our 20th wedding anniversary my wife and I will go on a romantic Caribbean cruise without the children.* You could go back and easily measure these objectives because they all answer the *who-will-do-how-much-of-what-by-when* question.

Crafting measurable objectives will help you meet your goals and ensure your success. Setting unrealistic goals or writing objectives that can't be measured set you up for failure. When you have goals that are too lofty or unrealistic, you will have a hard time meeting them, regardless of the objectives that accompany them.

Writing realistic goals with measurable objectives takes practice. It is a skill that you can learn at any point in your life and apply to improving any aspect of your sex life.

The following exercise, *Writing Values-Based Goals and Objectives,* will give you a framework for writing clear goals and measurable objectives. It will also help you examine how closely your goals reflect your values.

Acceptance and Commitment Exercise # 3: Writing Values-Based Goals and Objectives.

Instructions:

1. Pick one of the core sexual values that you identified in Chapter 11.

____

____

2. Describe how this value currently influences your sexual relationship with your partner.

____

____

____

____

3. Write one relationship goal that is related to this value.

____

____

____

____

4. Write three measurable objectives related to this goal.

____

____

____

Example:

Step 1. One of my core sexual values is:

Having a satisfying sexual relationship with my wife after twenty years of marriage.

Step 2. How this value currently influences my personal life:

Because I value having a satisfying sexual relationship with my wife, I try to balance my work and family responsibilities so they don't interfere with commitments I make to her. I will not stay late at work if we have something special planned. Because I travel often for work, when I am not on the road, I guard the time I have with my wife.

Step 3. One of my relationship goals is:

I would like to make love with my wife as often as possible.

Step 4. Three measurable objectives related to this goal are:

a. At least three times a week I will express my desire and availability to have sex with my wife.
b. Next month I will not schedule any work meetings or travel that conflicts with plans that my wife and I have made.
c. Next week I will send my wife a sexy text to let her know I still desire her sexually.

After you've set your goals and written your objectives, check back after the specified time period to see how you did. If you failed to meet a goal, it is okay if you decide to revise your time frames and add or delete objectives. While goals and objectives help give your life structure, they should also be flexible enough to adapt to change.

Some people think that setting goals and measurable objectives for things like having sex with your spouse is unrealistic and should be left alone to flow naturally. While there is validity to not planning *everything* in your life, your sex life is too important to be left entirely to chance. Try to think of your sexual goals and objectives as your *sexuality insurance.* It ensures that a day doesn't pass where you do not do something to strengthen your sexual relationship or enhance your personal sexual pleasure.

CHAPTER 13

Building Mindful Sexual Relationships

While there are several thing you can do to build a more mindful relationship, I'm going to focus on two things that fit well with our theme of sexual mindfulness: (1) developing grace and gratitude, and (2) communicating more effectively. They are two areas that are often overlooked in mindfulness training, yet contribute greatly to building a stronger sexual relationship with your partner.

Developing Grace and Gratitude

One of the most powerful ways to develop grace and gratitude towards your partner is through self-reflection. Self-reflection is a practice that goes back many centuries and has been practiced by adherents of most of the world's great religions.

Krech (2005) identifies four characteristics common to most forms of self-reflection: (1) scheduled practice time, (2) a quiet place, (3) questions to reflect on, and (4) a fearless moral self. To benefit from self-reflection you should practice it on a regular basis. Self-reflection can be done on a daily, weekly, or monthly basis. In a retreat setting, participants will often practice self-reflection more than once a day. Whatever the schedule, sticking to it is the key to making this practice part of your lifestyle. A quiet, secluded place that limits distraction is ideal.

Self-reflection revolves around answering questions that focus on your behavior towards other people. In this book they will focus on your partner. Self-reflection can be very painful when your actions towards your partner have not lived up to your moral and ethical standards. Self-reflection is designed to bring this to your attention and use it to become more grateful for your partner.

Naikan is a form of self-reflection that was developed in Japan by Ishin Yoskimoto in the 1940s. (Yoshimoto, 1973, Kreech, 2005). *Naikan* is a Japanese word that literally means "looking inside." The cornerstone of *Naikan* practice is the daily self-reflection on three questions that help you gain insight into and a deeper appreciation of your connectedness and indebtedness to others. *Naikan* practice also helps you develop a sense of grace and gratitude for other people and things that have contributed to your development.

The three questions are:

1. What have others done for me?
2. What have I done for others?
3. What problems have I caused others?

You can pick any issue related to your life or any person to focus these three questions on. For example, when I went to a Japanese Psychology retreat I did *Naikan* twice a day for ten days straight. I did it on my wife, mother, father, sons, co-workers and things such as my writing. In the case of my writing, I focused on all of the people and resources from my university that contributed to my success as a writer. I broke my life down into ten-year time frames and focused each meditation on what the person I focused on did for me during that time. It was exhausting and an emotional roller coaster, but well worth the effort. For our purposes I am going to ask you to do it on your partner going back as long as you have been together.

The daily self- reflection on the three questions focusing on your partner helps you gain insight into and a deeper appreciation of your connectedness and indebtedness to him/her. This forms the basis for the grace and the expression of gratitude that *Naikan* helps foster. Developing grace and becoming more grateful for what your partner has done for you shifts the focus from you and your "problems" to your partner, what they have done for you, and what problems you have caused them. In time, this shift results in you becoming more grateful and more connected to your partner.

Just imagine how this can benefit your relationship with your partner or spouse. Instead of being critical and ungrateful for the role she played in your happiness, success, and development, you turn this around and focus on how she enhanced your life and made it better. What would your relationship be like if you transformed this mindful insight into changes in your behavior? Imagine how your relationship might improve if you showed a little more grace and gratitude toward your partner every day.

Sexual Relationship Building Exercise # 1: Naikan Self-Reflection

Instructions:

1. Focus on your partner.
2. For the next week, spend 30 minutes (ten minutes on each question) each night reflecting on your partner by answering the following three questions:

    - What did I receive from my partner today?
    - What did I give to my partner today?
    - What troubles and difficulties did I cause my partner today?

3. Keep a brief diary in which you record your answers.
4. At the end of the week review your daily lists and write a thank-you note to your partner for something specific that she/he gave you or did for you.

Example:
Here is a sample from one of my clients that will give you a sense of the detail I'm talking about.

Focus: My husband

What my husband did for me this week:

1. He worked at his job 60 hours a week (almost 20 hours overtime).
2. He paid all the bills on time (wrote the checks, mailed the bills, balanced the checkbook; three hours a week, at least.
3. He changed the oil in the car.
4. He mowed the lawn on Sunday after church.
5. He weeded the flower beds.
6. He fixed my son's bicycle.
7. He drove my daughter to her soccer games on Saturday and Sunday so I could visit my sick mom.
8. He made the kids dinner on the days I had to visit my mom in the nursing home (3 nights a week).
9. He helped me figure out my mom's Medicare paperwork.
10. He comforted me when I was sad about my mom.
11. He rubbed my feet three times this week.
12. He gave me a couple of backrubs.
13. He made love with me three times despite the craziness of our schedules and all the overtime he had to work.
14. He walked the dog in the rain two nights after coming home late from work because I was helping the kids with their homework.
15. He came with me to church on Sunday even though it was his only day off and he is not religious.

What did I do for my husband?

1. I made him dinner on the nights I was not at the nursing home (4 dinners).
2. I washed his and the kids' clothes (2 loads each day).
3. I took care of the kids when he was working (5 days, 2 nights).
4. I listened to his problems at work when he came home.
5. I made love with him 3 times.

What problems did I cause my husband?

1. I was very sad about my mom and cried a lot when he was around.
2. I refused his offer for sex a few times when I knew he could have used it to relax.
3. I asked him to do more work around the house than he normally does, even though he worked 60 hours at his job.
4. I complained about the way the lawn and flower gardens looked and asked him to work on them on his only day off.
5. I asked him to go to church when I know he doesn't like going and feels out of place.
6. I told him I needed to buy a new dress for my friend's wedding and that we would need to pay for a hotel room to stay overnight because everyone was doing so.
7. I fell asleep a couple of nights instead of staying up and keeping him company after the kids went to sleep.
8. I made him miss his ball game on television on Sunday.

Self-reflection:

After doing this I reflected on how much more my husband did for me this week than I did for him and how he did this cheerfully, without my forcing him to do anything. He told me he loved me and was happy to help me.

You can see that doing *Naikan* on someone even for a week is a labor-intensive endeavor. You'll find that it's worth the time because this technique will help shift your attention—and your thinking—off yourself and onto your partner.

Strengthening Your Sexual Communication

Communication is the process by which you share information with your partner through words, symbols, signs, and behaviors. It includes spoken and written words as well as nonverbal messages such as gestures, facial expressions, and bodily messages or signals. Sexual communication poses unique challenges because of the difficulty of communicating in general, plus the personal nature of sexuality. Most of us haven't been raised in households where we are encouraged to talk about sex. Communicating effectively requires skill, patience, and commitment, as well as an understanding of sexual information.

Good communication is the foundation of healthy sexual relationships. Honest and accurate sexual communication is essential in developing and maintaining a good relationship with your partner. It is essential to obtaining sexual information for yourself as well as communicating information to your partner.

One of the things that makes it difficult to talk to your partner (especially new partners) about sex is the lack of a common sexual vocabulary. In the USA there is no uniform set of agreed-on words, phrases, and sexual language level that everyone agrees on. This makes it hard for you to be sure which words to use when trying to discuss a sexual issue with your partner.

Besides the actual words and phrases you use, your language level plays a big part in communicating with your partner about sex. There are four levels of language: childhood, street, everyday discourse, and scientific language.

1. Childhood language is simple, cute, and fun. Lovers have their own brand of childhood language. They may use it to describe their sexual anatomy and physiology, sexual desire, or need for pleasure. Pet names and phrases are part of this language.
2. Street language is tough, expressive, and emotional. Street language creates bonds between members of subcultures by sharing a language that members of mainstream society do not understand. It can also create barriers when lovers come from different cultures and do not share this bond.
3. Common discourse is the language level of mainstream society. It is comprised of words, expressions, and speech patterns that are neither intimate nor scientific. It is the language taught in schools and used in most communications.

4. Scientific/professional language is the discourse of the work world and professional community. It is the language that human sexuality professionals use to communicate with each other (Blonna and Carter, 2018).

Communication problems can occur when you and your partner use different language levels. This doesn't have to be a major problem, but it can get your discussion off on the wrong foot and sabotage your best intentions. For example, imagine that you would like to talk to your partner about your desire to have sex more often. You are quite comfortable using street language, but your partner is turned off by it and prefers to talk about sex using everyday or scientific language. Here is an example of how that conversation might play out.

> You: "I'd like to talk to you about our sex life."
>
> Her: "OK, what's on your mind?"
>
> You: "I feel like we don't fuck enough. I'd like to do it more often than we do."
>
> Her: "You are so disgusting. Do you always have to talk about sex in such a foul way?"
>
> You: "Huh, what do you mean?"
>
> Her: "I hate it when you use the word fuck. It is so cold. There is no love or intimacy in that word."

Obviously you could carry this dialogue on in a positive way and try to come to some form of a compromise, or it could lead to a blowup and both you getting mad at each other and shutting down. Agreeing on a language level is a good starting point for effective sexual communication.

There are three sets of skills that you can use to talk to your partner about sex: listening skills, observing skills, and responding skills (Blonna et al, 2011). I'll briefly go over them and give you lots of examples about how to use them with your partner.

Listening and Observing Skills

Getting your partner's full attention is pretty hard to do. In this era of multitasking, stand-up meetings, working lunches, drive-through everything, and incredibly full daily schedules, being able to sit with your partner and get his undivided attention is a luxury. The same holds true for your partner trying to get your undivided attention.

An easy way to conceptualize the building blocks of good listening is to use what I call the *Three V's and a B.* The three V's are verbals, vocals and visuals. The B stands for body language (Ivey et al, 1997a).

Verbals refers to two things: (1) the actual words you and your partner use when talking about sex, and (2) staying focused on what your partner is telling you (aka verbal tracking). As your partner speaks to you her words combine to form a dialogue that explains her point of view and tells her story. Staying focused on the words and the track the discussion is taking are equally important. Your mindfulness training will help you maintain this focus.

Keywords

Some of the words and short phrases are key to understanding the story and are therefore called keywords. Paying attention to the keywords is important. Here is an example:

> You: "That movie we saw was really erotic."
>
> Your Partner: "Yeah, especially the scenes in the *shower*. They really turned me on.
>
> *Shower* is the key word in that sentence. It would make sense for you to use it if you wanted to find out about what your partner found erotic about the shower.
>
> You: "Shower? What was erotic about the shower?"
>
> Your Partner: "The way they took their time and used the soap to lather each other and then get all of the right places nice and clean.

I could almost feel what that warmth and slipperiness was like."

Get the idea? Keywords tell the story because they capture the key thoughts and feelings inherent in the sentence.

Verbal tracking literally means following the track the discussion is taking. The goal of verbal tracking is to keep the dialogue going where your partner leads rather than cut it off and move it in the direction that you want to go in. This is a sure fire way to shut down the dialogue and show your partner that you really do not care about what she is saying. Let's use the shower dialogue as an example again. The original dialogue perfectly illustrates how to use verbal tracking simply by following the keyword , *shower.* The key word is the most important word in the sentence and captures the essence of what is being said.

You: "That movie we saw was really erotic."

Your Partner: " Yeah, especially the scenes in the *shower*. It really turned me on. "

You: "Shower? What was erotic about the shower?"

Your Partner: "The way they took their time and used the soap to lather each other and then get all of the right places nice and clean. I could almost feel what that warmth and slipperiness was like."

Following the keyword *shower* showed your partner that you were listening to her and wanted to know more. Imagine where the dialogue would have gone had you said this?

You: "That movie we saw was really erotic."

Your Partner: "Yeah, especially the scenes in the *shower*. They really turned me on."

You: "There is a really good new restaurant that just opened up in town. Want to go there tonight?"

Your Partner: "Restaurant? Didn't you hear anything I said about the shower part of the movie? You never listen to anything I have to say."

This is followed by your partner giving you a very annoyed look and reaching for the TV remote. Not only did you really show her you were not listening, you probably just blew your chance for a very erotic encounter in the shower with her.

Visuals refers to maintaining eye contact when your partner is talking. Maintaining eye contact with your partner is essential to good communication. It is especially important when your partner is speaking because it shows her that you are listening to and understanding her message. It also allows you to pick up on her nonverbal body language messages. We'll talk about body language a little later in the chapter.

Vocals refer to *how* words are spoken. Your voice is like an instrument that is capable of transmitting a broad range of tones. You and your partner transmit information by *how* you say things as much as *what* you actually say. If you listen carefully you'll notice that the pitch, volume, and speed of your partner's speech changes as she talks to you. These changes help you understand what is most important to her. When you are really communicating clearly you will vary the pitch, volume, and speed of your voice to match hers. This shows her that you are really listening with understanding.

For instance, your partner might lower her pitch and volume when dealing with sensitive information that evokes strong feelings in her. She might slow the pace, use frequent pauses, and intersperse her words with sighs and shallow breaths. This pattern of speaking and breathing sends a distinct message regarding her feeling very vulnerable discussing the information.

When you are really listening with understanding you will see and hear this and adjust your own vocal qualities to match this. By matching your partner's pitch, volume, and pace, you show her that you hear and feel what she is saying. Once again, this is where your mindfulness training comes in handy. If you've been meditating and being more mindful this will automatically carry over into paying more attention to the nuances in the vocal tone of your partner.

Nonverbal Communication

There are many ways to convey sexual information nonverbally through your body language, gestures, and movements. Nonverbal communication can transmit sexual messages as effectively, and in some cases more effectively than verbal techniques.

Body language describes the nonverbal messages you send through your posture, gestures, and movement. You demonstrate positive, or open, body language by having a relaxed posture, steady eye contact, nods of your head, and an occasional smile or happy expression. These tell your partner that you are approachable and receptive. You show negative, or closed, body language with visible signs of tension such as having clenched fists or tight jaw muscles, a closed posture (your arms folded and your body shifted sideways and the like), and facial expressions ranging from anger to disbelief. Negative body language shows that you are either apathetic or disturbed about something your partner just said. You can use this information in two ways when talking about sex with your partner.

- You can be mindful of your own body language and be sure to show an open, receptive posture.
- You can sense your partner's level of acceptance or rejection and use this information to gently confront your partner and clear things up.

We'll talk about using gentle confrontation when we get to the responding part of this chapter a little later.

Understanding Silence and Time Differentials

Time means different things to different people. Thirty seconds of silence in the middle of a sentence might seem like an eternity to you but very reasonable to your partner. Your partner might need extra time to formulate his thoughts about something you just said, especially if it related to a sexual topic that he is uncomfortable or unfamiliar with. Silence does not have to be perceived as a sign of a breakdown in communication. Silence is a necessary part of effective communication that is often overlooked. You and your partner need time to listen, digest, and understand sexual messages. Silence allows you and your partner time to reflect as you formulate your thoughts and words.

Many people often have a hard time dealing with silence in relationships because they perceive even short periods of quiet time as "endless" or "interminable." Becoming more accepting of silence is a major skill in listening with understanding. One of the things you learn when you practice mindfulness meditation is how relative time is. In the beginning you probably thought that just sitting still for 15-30 minutes would seem like an eternity. Now you find that 15 or 30 minutes passes quickly and catches you by surprise. This is a big advantage when understanding what time means to your partner and how much time he needs to gather his thoughts and explain himself.

Touch is an extremely important form of nonverbal sexual communication. A reassuring touch on the arm, a gentle squeeze, a subtle placement of the hand where you want to be touched all speak volumes without uttering a single word.

If you have a hard time asking for something specific because the words are hard to say, try saying them by using your body to convey the message. You can send messages regarding where, how hard, how fast, and how often you want to be stimulated without saying anything. Putting your hand on your partner's hand or hip and guiding them or moving your body a certain way can allow you to control the action without saying anything. There is no right or wrong way to do this. You just need to experiment with your partner and establish your own guidelines.

Six Better Listening Tips

1. **Keep yourself in good mental and physical shape**. Good communication takes time and energy. When you are too tired, your energy level is low and you simply don't have the energy to think clearly and communicate well.
2. **Maintain eye contact when your partner is speaking**. This will assure him that what he is saying is being heard.
3. **Listen actively rather than passively.** Use body language to reflect what your partner is saying. Nod in agreement, smile, or laugh at her humor.
4. **Avoid distracting mannerisms.** Things such as hair twirling, fingernail inspecting, checking text messages, or glancing at the television are disrespectful and show boredom or disinterest.
5. **Use paraphrasing when you don't understand something.** Use paraphrasing (repeating what the other person has said, in your own words), to convey understanding. Tell the person, " I think this is what you said," then paraphrase their statement. Follow it up with a check-out question like, "Is that right?"
6. **Use Your Mindfulness Training to Keep Your Mind from Wandering**. It's easy to get distracted because you can listen and think much faster than your partner can speak. Make your partner feel that she is the only person in the world at that moment.

Responding Skills

A conversation is a two-way dialogue. This means that your feedback is as important as your partner's statements in moving the discussion along. There are several responding skills you can use to provide feedback to your partner.

Minimal encouragers are techniques that work by using the "minimum" amount of feedback necessary to encourage your partner to keep talking. Minimal encouragers can be either nonverbal or verbal. Verbal and nonverbal encouragers are often used together (Ivey et al, 1997a). For instance, you might combine a head nod or hand gesture with a key word from what your partner said.

Nonverbal minimal encouragers include the following: (1) relaxed, open body language, (2) facial expressions (nods, eyes, smile, eyebrows, etc.), and (3) hand gestures (roll hands to indicate "continue"). As I mentioned previously, a relaxed, open body posture alone will encourage your partner to talk by setting an accepting, inviting tone. Encouraging facial gestures include smiling, arching your eyebrows, and nodding or tilting your head. These nonverbal gestures indicate that you hear what your partner is saying, and want him to continue. Turning your hands over (rolling) indicates that you want him to continue. This simple, nonverbal gesture alone can keep your partner talking and encourage him to go into greater detail on a subject (Ivey et al, 1997a).

Verbal Minimal Encouragers include minimal verbal utterances such as "Ummm" or "Uh -huh," and repeating key words without any additional dialogue. The idea is to keep your speaking to a minimum and let your partner do most of the talking. Simple "Ummms" and "Uh-huhs" show your partner that you are paying attention and understand what he is saying. Repeating key words is a simple way to get your partner to expand on words and themes contained in what he just told you without asking him a bunch of direct questions. You'll see in the next section why just asking questions is not the best approach (Ivey et al, 1997a).

Questioning is by far the most common way of getting your partner to explain herself in greater detail. Questions serve a variety of functions. Here are a couple of positive and negative things to consider when asking *sexual questions.*

Positive Uses of Questioning

1. Questions are a good way to start a conversation. Questions can be used to start a new conversation. They shift the focus of the

conversation off of you and onto your partner. Open questions such as, "What did you want to talk to me about?" or "What would you like to talk about?" are examples of open questions used to start a conversation.

2. Questions can help enrich, elaborate, and bring out specific details about something your partner said that you want her to expand upon. Questions such as, " Can you give me a specific example of what you meant by …" are a way of asking for specific details.

Potential Problems with Questioning

1. Questioning Shifts the Focus Off of Yourself and Onto Your Partner.

While it can be a good thing to get your partner talking by asking him a question, asking too many questions can be viewed as an attempt to avoid having to share your own thoughts and feelings about the issue. You need to make sure that you don't use questions for this purpose.

2. Questions can Foster Mistrust.

Because questions place the direction (and therefore the power) of the interview in your hands you need to use them judiciously. Using too many questions together and too early in a discussion will create mistrust. Your partner will wonder why this is all about her and your questions can be viewed as blaming her for the problem or miscommunication.

3. *Why* questions can put your partner on the defensive.

When you use *why* questions honestly and in moderation, they can help your partner search for the reasons behind her statements and actions. *Why* questions, however, can also put her on the defensive. Your partner might perceive questions such as "Why did you do that?", "Why do you think that?", or "Why do you feel that way?" as forms of attack. She may feel that you are asking her to justify her thoughts and feelings and she may go on the defensive because of this. Lastly, *why* questions are usually unanswerable (Ivey et al, 1997a).

Something to Think About: Try to Avoid Asking *Why* Questions. I always have a good time talking about *why* questions with my students and clients. I usually go a little crazy, raise my voice, and storm around the room spouting off the following litany to really hammer home my point:

"You ask me WHY I think and feel that way. Well, here's why... The reason I feel or think anything at any given point in space and time is a result of the following factors: my genetic inheritance, cultural upbringing, educational level, socioeconomic status, the number of hours I slept the night before, my nutritional status, level of fitness, the nature of my relationship, the last time I had an orgasm, my use of psychoactive substances in the past 24 hours, my memory, the interaction of all of these factors, and a host of OTHER factors too numerous to list. In short, who the hell knows WHY I feel, think, or behave the way I do."

It is much more productive to ask *what* and *how* questions when seeking clarification. Your partner can describe *what* he is thinking and feeling and *how* he would prefer to feel, think and behave. It is much more productive and less threatening to focus on these issues. You can get the same information you seek and help create the same insights by asking what and how questions.

Open-Ended Statements and Questions

The best way to get your partner to clarify what he is saying is to use open-ended statements and questions. Open-ended statements are queries that cannot be answered with a simple yes or no. To answer them, your partner ***must*** go into detail. That is why they are excellent for initiating a dialogue—because they cannot be answered with a simple yes/no response. I prefer to use the word *statements*, rather than questions, because these queries do not end with a question mark.

Examples of open-ended statements:

"Tell me more about that."
"Describe that in more detail for me please."
"Explain how you feel about that."
"Clarify that for me a little more."
"Expand on that a little more."

Open-ended questions are similar to statements except that they end with a question mark. They are often referred to as open-direct questions because of this. They generally fall into the who, what, when, where, and why, categories.

Examples of Open Ended Questions
"What did you do then?"
"How did you feel after that?"
"When did all of this happen?"
"Where were you going when this happened?"
"Why do you think you were singled out for this?" (Use this type sparingly, if at all.)

A separate category of open-ended questions are called *permission-asking questions* because they end in a question mark and are asked in such a way that your partner perceives that she is being asked permission to explore these sensitive, potentially distressing areas. If asked in a respectful, gentle way, your partner will usually respond with detailed answers, even though they technically could answer this type of question with a yes/no response.

Examples of permission-asking open questions:
"Could you please explain that more fully?"
"Can you please give me another example of that?"
"Could you go over that one more time for me, please?"

Closed, or Yes/No Questions

Closed questions are queries that can be answered yes or no and typically don't prompt your partner to give you a detailed response. They are the weakest way to initiate a conversation or clarify an issue. I would recommend either not using them at all or keeping them to a bare minimum when talking about sex with your partner.

Sexual Relationship Building Exercise # 1: Using Open-Ended Statements

Purpose: The purpose of this exercise is to help you become more mindful of using open-ended statements whenever you are unclear about something your partner says to you. It will help you get used to seeking clarification and clearing up miscommunications before they can fester and cause problems in the bedroom.

Instructions:

1. This week start becoming more mindful of unclear statements that your partner makes that you do not understand.
2. Pick a statement and, in a gentle way, confront your partner as soon as the miscommunication occurs.
3. Use "I" language by taking responsibility for the misunderstanding by saying something such as, "I'm really not sure what that means. Please ....", or "I'm having a hard time understanding that, can you please...?"
4. After your "I" language introduction use one of the following open-ended statements to finish the sentence and clear things up:

    - "Please tell me more."
    - "Tell me how you feel about that."
    - "Tell me what are your thoughts about that."
    - "Please explain that in greater detail."

- "Tell me a little more about that."
- "Please give me an example of what you mean."

5. When you are done, write these gentle confrontations down and examine how your efforts to clear up the miscommunication went.

With practice, you will become more aware of miscommunications and take more responsibility for clearing them up. The following ideas can help you develop your listening skills.

Paraphrasing

Paraphrasing is one of the strongest responding skills you can use when talking about sex with your partner. Paraphrasing does the following things:

- It shows your partner you are listening carefully.
- It demonstrates how much you really understand about what your partner just said.
- It gives you a chance to clarify issues that are still unclear.

Effective paraphrases include three elements;

- A shortened restatement of what your partner said using your own words.
- The use of a key word from what your partner told you.
- The use of a "check it out" phrase (Ivey et al, 1997a).

Here is an example of paraphrasing, using the shower scene from earlier in the chapter:

> Your Partner: "That movie last night was very erotic. That scene in the shower was a real turn-on. When he was washing her in the shower I got very turned on. When he was lathering his hands and then spreading that hot soapy water all over her body I started to get hot. It is a

good thing we were in the movies and not home. I think I would have put the video on pause if we were home."

You: (Restatement in your own words): "Wow, that shower scene really seemed to have an effect on you."

You (Keyword/Phrase): "It really turned you on."

You (Check Out): "Am I right?"

Your partner: "Absolutely. Want to go take a shower with me right now?"

Paraphrasing not only shows your partner that you hear what she is saying and understand it, but it also gives her the opportunity to let you know if your take on things is accurate or not.

Confronting Discrepancies

If you are listening and observing carefully you will often pick up on discrepancies or mixed messages. For example imagine that you ask your partner to try some new sexual activity and he says, "Sure, no problem." Unfortunately the *way* he said it indicated that there *was* a problem. He didn't make eye contact, folded his arms across his chest, and said it in a way that seemed disingenuous. Now what do you do? How do you respond?

The bottom line is that if you sense there is a problem or miscommunication because of a mixed message, it is *your responsibility* to clear it up. *You* are the one with the problem, not your partner. You are the one who is unclear about the message or his intentions in sending it. In his mind there might not be any problem and since he sent the message he might not even sense that he sent you a mixed message.

A simple way to clear up discrepancies and miscommunications is to use gentle confrontation. Most people are uncomfortable with the thought of **confrontation**. When asked to free-associate about the term confrontation, most of the students and clients I've worked with typically say things such as, "fight," "anger," strong disagreement," "agitation," " stress," "catch someone at something," "call someone on something." Most of the associations are negative. If you are like most of the people I've worked with you'll probably have to rethink your assumptions about confrontation before you can begin to use it effectively.

To do this, you need to redefine confrontation as "supportive challenge." Rather than view confrontation as a harsh "going against" your partner, it can be viewed as a gentle "going with" your partner by seeking her help in clarifying any **discrepancies, incongruities**, or **mixed messages** in her story. You do this by gently and respectfully pointing out discrepancies in your partner's story and asking for clarification.

Ivey et al (1997b) recommends a "two-handed" approach to confrontation. This approach combines body language with words to identify discrepancies, incongruities and mixed messages in what your partner said. Here are simple instructions on how to use this highly effective technique.

1. Look your partner in the eye, call her by her name, and put the confrontation in a gentle, supportive context.

"Doris, I know this is difficult for you to talk about and I want to understand what you are saying, but something about what you just said troubles me."

Use the "first hand." Introduce the discrepancy by extending one hand as you speak.

"On the one hand, you stated that you found the shower scene in the movie a real turn on."

Use the "second hand." Leave the first hand extended and extend your other hand as you continue the description.

"But on the other hand when I've suggested sex in the shower or the bathtub you weren't very receptive."

Finish with a gentle, probing, open-ended clarifying statement.

"Can you please explain this to me?"

Using a two-handed approach is easy to remember, uses body language to reinforce the gentle confrontation, and provides a simple framework for you to clear up discrepancies in your sexual communication.

There are many more ways to improve your sexual communication, but if you can use the simple examples in this chapter you will have a great start on communicating more effectively. Your mindfulness training will really help you identify barriers in your communication and allow you to resolve them before they become major problems.

The following exercise is a simple assessment form to help you gauge how well you communicate with your partner.

Mindfulness and Assertiveness

Becoming more mindful of your assertiveness (or lack thereof) will help you develop and maintain a more equal relationship and co-exist with your partner in a respectful way. In order to do this you must be clear about the similarities and differences between assertiveness, aggressiveness, and non-assertiveness.

Assertiveness is often confused with aggressiveness. Many people think that assertiveness and aggressiveness are the same thing. In actuality, assertiveness is not a negative attribute. It is based on mutual respect and democracy in relationships. Assertiveness is understanding your wants and needs and pursuing them without infringing on the wants and needs of others. Aggressiveness, by contrast, is pursuing your needs and wants without any regard to how this affects the rights of others. Often, aggressive people get their needs met at the expense of others. Nonassertiveness is failing to pursue your needs and wants while allowing others to meet theirs.

Lack of assertiveness is a key factor in doing things that conflict with your values and that you don't want to do. When you are nonassertive and continue to get taken advantage of by your partner, it fills you with resentment and hostility. Needless to say, these are not the kinds of feelings that foster great sex. In an attempt to avoid conflict, when you act nonassertively, you'll say yes to something when you really want to say no. This temporarily relieves you from feeling guilty, but unfortunately, it causes you to get trapped into doing things you really do not want to do. When this happens, you begin to feel miserable because you've lost control of your life and your time. This simple exercise on how to say no can help you begin to assert yourself when your partner tries to corner you into doing something you really do not want to do.

Sexual Relationship Building Exercise # 3: How to Say No

Purpose: Saying no is not always easy, but it is essential if you are to be assertive and communicate your desires more clearly. The following are clear guidelines for saying no.

Instructions:

1. Face your partner from a normal distance (about 3 feet).
    - If you are too far away, you may appear timid.
    - If you crowd your partner, you border on being aggressive.
2. Look him directly in the eye.
    - Averting eye contact is a sure giveaway that you will cave in.
3. Keep your head up and your body relaxed.
    - Don't be a shrinking violet.
4. Speak clearly, firmly, and at a volume that can be heard.

5. Just say "no."
    - You do not need to clarify why.
6. Be prepared to repeat it.
    - Sometimes your partner will be persistent.
7. Stick to your guns.
    - Do not give in—it gets easier with practice.

If you feel a need to explain why you are declining, here are a few tips for setting the stage:

1. Thank your partner for the offer.
2. Express your appreciation.
3. Affirm your love.
4. Reject the offer, not your partner.

Example: Your Partner Wants You to Go Over His Friend's House and Sit in The Hot Tub With His Friend and His Wife

> Husband: John and Sara asked us to go over to their place at 8:00pm and drink a little wine and sit in their hot tub.
>
> You: "Thanks for thinking of me before saying yes or no to John and Sara." (thank you)
>
> "I really appreciate the way you like to keep in contact with your friends and try new things." (express appreciation)
>
> "John, you know I love you and will do most anything you want." (express your love)
>
> "However, I am going to decline. I really am uncomfortable being in a hot tub with another couple." (reject the offer)

Assertiveness begins with understanding your values, goals, and commitments. You've already done that hard work so now you are ready to assert yourself. Practice being assertive in the mirror. Come up with a list of common examples where your partner has taken advantage of you in the past and use them for practice. You can also practice with unsolicited telephone offers. This is often easier because you do not have to look the caller in the eyes.

Sexual Communication Exercise # 3: Sexual Communication Satisfaction Questionnaire

Purpose: This questionnaire assesses your satisfaction with your sexual communication with your partner.

Instructions: Use the following scale to indicate how strongly you agree or disagree with each statement:

5 Strongly agree 4 Agree 3 Neither agree nor disagree 2 Disagree 1 Strongly Disagree

1. I tell my partner when I am especially sexually satisfied.
2. I am satisfied with my partner's ability to communicate his/her sexual desires to me.
3. I do not let my partner know things that I find pleasing during sex.
4. I am very satisfied with the quality of our sexual interactions.
5. I do not hesitate to let my partner know when I want to have sex with him/her.
6. I do not tell my partner whether or not I am sexually satisfied.
7. I am dissatisfied over the degree to which my partner and I discuss our sexual relationship.
8. I am not afraid to show my partner what kind of sexual behavior I find satisfying.

9. I would not hesitate to show my partner what is a sexual turn-on to me.
10. My partner does not show me when he/she is sexually satisfied.
11. I show my partner what pleases me during sex.
12. I am displeased with the manner in which my partner and I communicate with each other during sex.
13. My partner does not show me things he/she finds pleasing during sex.
14. I show my partner when I am sexually satisfied.
15. My partner does not let me know whether sex has been satisfying or not.
16. I do not show my partner when I am sexually satisfied.
17. I am satisfied concerning my ability to communicate about sexual matters with my partner.
18. My partner shows me by the way he/she touches me if he/she is satisfied.
19. I am dissatisfied with my partner's ability to communicate his/her sexual desire to me.
20. I have no way of knowing when my partner is sexually satisfied.
21. I am not satisfied in the majority of our sexual interactions.
22. I am pleased with the manner in which my partner and I communicate with each other after sex.

There is no correct score. This is just designed to give you more information about your level of communication. Have your partner take it and then compare notes (Blonna and Carter, 2018).

CHAPTER 14

Mindful Massage

Massage is one of the greatest sensual delights you can share with your partner. Massage can be a stand-alone sensual activity or a prelude to sexual intercourse. Massage allows you to explore every nook and cranny of your partner's body in a relaxed, sensual way. Devoting your full attention to kneading, stroking, and manipulating your partner's body requires you to be fully mindful of the present moment.

Giving a massage is an excellent training tool for mindfulness. All of your senses are involved in giving a massage. Primary among them is the sense of touch. When you give a massage, you must be acutely aware of pressure and motion and the feel of your muscles as well as your partner's skin and flesh. Your sense of smell gets involved because of the natural scent of your partner's skin, hair, and body fluids. Also, many of the massage oils commonly used are scented and can add an extra olfactory dimension to your experience. Visually, you are focused on the shape and contour of your partner's body as your hands move along the ridges and lines of her muscles. The only sense that isn't automatically involved in giving a massage is taste, but with a little creativity on your part you can even work that in.

You can give full-body or partial massages. Sometimes just a back massage or a foot massage will do the trick. At other times, a full-body massage, complete with scented candles, is preferred. Massage can be a prelude to other forms of sexual activity. In sensual massage, the focus shifts to providing more direct contact with the genitals and other erogenous zones. In this case massage blends with masturbation if you want to transform it into an experience capable of leading to orgasm. The focus of your ministrations shifts to the genitals and other erogenous zones.

Mindful Massage Exercise # 1: Mindful Foot Massage

Purpose: This activity is designed to help you start to apply your mindfulness training to sexual activities with your partner. Learning how to give your partner's feet 100% of your attention without judgment sets the stage for doing the same thing with your partner's genitals and full body during other erotic activities.

The following is a set of preliminary instructions to use for all of the mindful sex activities.

1. Read all of the instructions for whatever mindful sex activity you choose to engage in before doing it with your partner.
2. This will ensure that there are no surprises and you are comfortable with the instructions.
3. Allow 30 minutes of uninterrupted time for each activity.
4. Do this and all of the other mindful sex activities in the bedroom on your own bed.
5. Make sure the room is at a temperature that you and your partner find relaxing.
6. Put relaxing background music on that will help cancel out distracting sounds from the outside environment.
7. Make sure that the music you choose is instrumental and has no singing. Songs tend to distract your mind and take the focus off of the activity and onto thinking about the music.
8. Turn off your cell phone, television, and any distracting device.
9. Burn your favorite scented candle or incense.
10. Take a shower or bath with your partner before engaging in any of these activities.
11. Be mindful of the warmth of the water, the smell and feel of your partner and the soap as you move it over your partner's body and get clean and ready for these mindful sex activities.

12. When performing this activity keep your mind on your partner's body. Focus your attention on what each motion feels like and how your partner responds to your actions.
13. When your mind drifts to the past or future, or starts "thinking" or "worrying" about if you are doing things right or perfect, just get back to noticing, without judgment, what each motion feels like and how your partner responds to your actions.
14. Whenever your mind drifts, say to yourself, *there goes my runaway mind again, taking me out of the present moment*, and shift your focus back on what you are doing to your partner.

That's it for general instructions. I will talk you through each activity, step by step. Relax and enjoy the process.

Specific Instructions

1. Make sure you have read and followed the general instructions.
2. Have your partner lie face down on the bed with his or her feet extending over the edge of the bed about 12 inches.
3. Pull up a stool or chair and position it so that your partner's feet are directly in front of you and you can grasp them easily while seated.
4. Spend a few moments just noticing your partner's feet with all five of your senses.
5. Get close and examine each foot carefully. Imagine you are a scientist, taking notice of the size, shape, color, texture, and weight of your partner's feet.

PAUSE A FEW SECONDS

6. Now close your eyes and examine your partner's feet using your senses of touch, smell, and taste.

7. Use your nose, cheeks, face, head, and hair to examine your partner's feet.

PAUSE A FEW SECONDS

8. Now take a quick taste. You just washed your partner's feet so they are clean. Suck on a toe, lick your partner's instep, heel, or achilles tendon. You don't have to get too freaky— just take a taste.

PAUSE A FEW SECONDS

Notice your thoughts, self-talk, mental images and emotions about experiencing your partner's feet with all five of your senses.

If your mind wanders into the future or the past or fills with unhelpful thoughts and feelings, note that this is happening and say to yourself, *there goes my runaway mind again, taking me out of the present moment*, and focus on your partner's feet.

9. Spread oil or powder all over your partner's feet and ankles.
10. Take your time and rub it all over, making sure to get between your partner's toes.
11. Notice how the oil or powder feels and smells as you rub it into your partner's feet.

PAUSE A FEW SECONDS

12. Rub any excess over your partner's legs all the way up to your partner's buttocks.
13. Now stand and cradle both of your partner's feet in your two hands.
14. Notice the weight and feel of your partner's feet in your hands.
15. Press your partner's feet against your genitals.

16. If you are a woman, notice the sensations in your genitals as you press your partner's feet against your vulva.
17. If you are a man, have your partner's feet cradle around your penis and feel the soles of your partner's feet against your scrotum.
18. Notice the sensations in your penis and scrotum as you press your partner's feet against them.

PAUSE A FEW SECONDS

19. Let your partner know how good this feels.

Notice your thoughts, self-talk, mental images and emotions as you press your partners feet against your genitals.

If your mind wanders into the future or the past or fills with unhelpful thoughts and feelings note that this is happening and say to yourself, *there goes my runaway mind again, taking me out of the present moment*, and focus on your partner's feet and the sensations in your genitals.

PAUSE A FEW SECONDS

20. Now sit back down and shift your focus off of yourself and back on your partner's feet.
21. Start at your partner's ankles.
22. Grasp both feet at the ankle and pull your hands back towards you as you slide your thumbs over the heels and down the center of your partner's feet.
23. Apply pressure with your thumbs as you pull your hands along the center of your partner's feet.
24. Do this several times.

PAUSE A FEW SECONDS

25. Now shift your focus to your partner's left foot.

26. Start at your partner's left ankle and while grasping your partner's left foot at the ankle with both of your hands, pull your hands back towards you as you slide your thumbs over the heel and down the center of your partner's left foot.
27. Apply pressure with your thumbs as you pull your hands along the center of your partner's left foot.
28. Do this several times.

PAUSE A FEW SECONDS

29. Now shift your focus to the toes on your partner's left foot.
30. Start with the big toe and using just your thumb and forefinger, gently pull and twist the big toe. Use extra oil or powder to make them very slippery.
31. Repeat this action a couple of times on the big toe.

PAUSE A FEW SECONDS

32. Work your way down to the next toe and as you do this, roll your finger between the toes and focus on the area between your partner's toes.
33. Now using just your thumb and forefinger, gently pull and twist the next toe. Use extra oil or powder to make them very slippery.
34. Repeat this action a couple of times on the second toe.

PAUSE A FEW SECONDS

35. Work your way down to the middle toe and as you do this, roll your finger between the toes and focus on the area between your partner's toes.
36. Now using just your thumb and forefinger, gently pull and twist the middle toe. Use extra oil or powder to make them very slippery.
37. Repeat this action a couple of times on the middle toe.

PAUSE A FEW SECONDS

38. Work your way down to the next toe and as you do this, roll your finger between the toes and focus on the area between your partner's toes.
39. Now using just your thumb and forefinger, gently pull and twist the next toe. Use extra oil or powder to make them very slippery.
40. Repeat this action a couple of times on the next toe.

PAUSE A FEW SECONDS

41. Work your way down to the pinkie toe and as you do this, roll your finger between the toes and focus on the area between your partner's toes.
42. Now using just your thumb and forefinger, gently pull and twist the pinkie toe. Use extra oil or powder to make them very slippery.
43. Repeat this action a couple of times on the pinkie toe.

PAUSE A FEW SECONDS

Notice your thoughts, self-talk, mental images and emotions as you massage your partner's foot and toes.

If your mind wanders into the future or the past or fills with unhelpful thoughts and feelings, note that this is happening and say to yourself, *there goes my runaway mind again, taking me out of the present moment*, and focus on your partner's body and the sensations in your hands and fingers as you massage.

44. Now focus on the arch in your partner's left foot.
45. Grab your partner's foot with both hands and use your thumbs to knead just the arch.
46. Repeat this action a couple of times.

PAUSE A FEW SECONDS

47. When you are finished kneading it with your thumbs for a few times, shift and use your fist to rub it in a circular motion, putting more pressure on it than before.
48. Repeat this action a couple of times.

PAUSE A FEW SECONDS

49. Now grasp all of the toes in your partner's left foot with one hand and rotate them in a circular motion.
50. As you continue to hold all of the toes on your partner's left foot in one hand, push the ball of your partner's foot down towards the floor while gently pulling your partner's left heel back towards you with the other hand. This will gently stretch your partner's entire left foot.
51. Do this a couple of times.

PAUSE A FEW SECONDS

52. You are now ready to shift to the right foot.
53. Stand up and leaning over, spread more oil on your partner's legs, behind the knees, and buttocks.
54. Notice the shape, smell, feel, and taste of your partner's legs and buttocks as you make your way up your partner's left leg, over the buttocks, and down the right leg to the right foot.
55. Take time to nuzzle your partner's legs and buttocks.

PAUSE A FEW SECONDS

56. Work your way to the right foot by sliding your hands up your partner's left leg, over their buttocks, and down the right leg all the way to the ankle.
57. As you move up one leg, over the buttocks, and down the next leg, press and knead the areas you go over.

PAUSE A FEW SECONDS

58. Now shift your focus to your partner's right foot.
59. Start at your partner's right ankle, and while grasping your partner's right foot in both of your hands, pull them back over the heel and down the center of your partner's foot.
60. Apply pressure with your thumbs as you pull your hands along the center of your partner's right foot.
61. Do this several times.

PAUSE A FEW SECONDS

62. Now shift your focus to the toes on your partner's right foot.
63. Start with the big toe and using just your thumb and forefinger, gently pull and twist the big toe.
64. Use extra oil or powder to make it very slippery.
65. Repeat this action a couple of times on the big toe.

PAUSE A FEW SECONDS

Notice your thoughts, self-talk, mental images and emotions as you massage your partner's toes.

If your mind wanders into the future or the past or fills with unhelpful thoughts and feelings, note that this is happening and say to yourself, *there goes my runaway mind again, taking me out of the present moment*, and focus on your partner's body and the sensations in your hands and fingers as you massage your partner's toes.

66. Work your way down to the next toe and as you do this, roll your finger between the toes and focus on the area between your partner's toes.
67. Now using just your thumb and forefinger, gently pull and twist the next toe.
68. Use extra oil or powder to make them very slippery.
69. Repeat this action a couple of times on the second toe.

PAUSE A FEW SECONDS

70. Work your way down to the middle toe, and as you do this, roll your finger between the toes and focus on the area between your partner's toes.
71. Now, using just your thumb and forefinger, gently pull and twist the middle toe.
72. Use extra oil or powder to make them very slippery.
73. Repeat this action a couple of times on the middle toe.

PAUSE A FEW SECONDS

74. Work your way down to the next toe, and as you do this, roll your finger between the toes and focus on the area between your partner's toes.
75. Now, using just your thumb and forefinger, gently pull and twist the next toe.
76. Use extra oil or powder to make them very slippery.
77. Repeat this action a couple of times on the next toe.

PAUSE A FEW SECONDS

78. Work your way down to the pinkie toe, and as you do this, roll your finger between the toes and focus on the area between your partner's toes.
79. Now, using just your thumb and forefinger, gently pull and twist the pinkie toe.
80. Use extra oil or powder to make them very slippery.
81. Repeat this action a couple of times on the pinkie toe.

PAUSE A FEW SECONDS

82. Now focus on the arch in your partner's right foot.

83. Grab your partner's foot with both hands and use your thumbs to knead just the arch.
84. Repeat this action a couple of times.

PAUSE A FEW SECONDS

85. When you are finished kneading it with your thumbs for a few times, shift and use your fist to rub it in a circular motion, putting more pressure on it than before.
86. Repeat this action a couple of times.

PAUSE A FEW SECONDS

87. Now grasp all of the toes in your partner's right foot with one hand and rotate them in a circular motion.
88. As you continue to hold all of the toes on your partner's right foot in one hand, push the ball of the foot down towards the floor while gently pulling your partner's right heel towards you with the other hand.
89. Do this a couple of times.

PAUSE A FEW SECONDS

90. Gently wipe off the excess oil from your partner's feet and legs and cover them with a blanket or towel.
91. Let your partner relax and enjoy the warmth and peacefulness.

Notice your thoughts, self-talk, mental images and emotions as you lie quietly next to your partner for a few moments.

If your mind wanders into the future or the past or fills with unhelpful thoughts and feelings, note that this is happening and say to yourself, *there goes my runaway mind again, taking me out of the present moment*, and focus on your partner's body and the sensations in your hands and fingers as you relax and lie next to your partner.

Mindful Massage Exercise # 2: Mindful Back Massage

Purpose: This activity is designed to build upon your mindful sexuality training by shifting your focus onto giving a back massage. Learning how to give your partner's neck, shoulders, back, and buttocks 100% of your attention without judgment sets the stage for doing the same thing with your partner's genitals and full body during other erotic activities.

The following is a set of preliminary instructions to use for all of the mindful sex activities.

1. Read all of the instructions for whatever mindful sex activity you choose to engage in before doing it with your partner.
2. This will ensure that there are no surprises and you are comfortable with the instructions.
3. Allow 30 minutes of uninterrupted time for each activity.
4. Do this and all of the other mindful sex activities in the bedroom on your own bed.
5. Make sure the room is at a temperature that you and your partner find relaxing.
6. Put relaxing background music on that will help cancel out distracting sounds from the outside environment.
7. Make sure that the music you choose is instrumental and has no singing. Songs tend to distract your mind and take the focus off of the activity and onto thinking about the music.
8. Turn off your cell phone, television, and any distracting device.
9. Burn your favorite scented candle or incense.
10. Take a shower or bath with your partner before engaging in any of these activities.
11. Be mindful of the warmth of the water, the smell and feel of your partner and the soap as you move it over your partner's body and get clean and ready for these mindful sex activities.

12. When performing this activity keep your mind on your partner's body. Focus your attention on what each motion feels like and how your partner responds to your actions.
13. When your mind drifts to the past or future, or starts "thinking" or "worrying" about if you are doings things right or perfect, just get back to noticing, without judgment, what each motion feels like and how your partner responds to your actions.
14. Whenever your mind drifts, say to yourself, *there goes my runaway mind again taking me out of the present moment*, and shift your focus back on what you are doing to your partner.

That's it for general instructions. I will talk you through each activity, step by step. Relax and enjoy the process.

Specific Instructions:

Before following these instructions, make sure that you have read the preliminary instructions.

1. Have your partner lie on their stomach with their head pointing towards the head of the bed.
2. Have them move down so their head is about 16" from the end of the bed. Their feet and ankles will hang over the end of the bed.
3. Spend a few moments just noticing your partner's back with all five of your senses.
4. Get close and examine your partner's back from top to bottom. Imagine you are a scientist, taking note of the size, shape, color, texture, and taste of your partner's back.

PAUSE A FEW SECONDS

5. Now close your eyes and examine your partner's back from neck to buttocks using your senses of touch, smell, and taste.

6. Use your nose, cheeks, face, head, and hair to examine your partner's back.

PAUSE A FEW SECONDS

Now take a quick taste. You just washed your partner's back so it is clean. Suck or lick any part of your partner's back. You don't have to get too freaky—just take a taste.

PAUSE A FEW SECONDS

Notice your thoughts, self-talk, mental images, and emotions about experiencing your partner's back with all five of your senses.

If your mind wanders into the future or the past or fills with unhelpful thoughts and feelings, note that this is happening and say to yourself, *there goes my runaway mind again, taking me out of the present moment*, and focus on your partner's back.

7. Kneel on the bed with your toes curled under you and at the very end of the mattress. You can kneel on a pillow or put it under your buttocks if it makes you more comfortable.
8. Position yourself so your partner's head is directly in front of your genitals.
9. Your partner's arms should be extended forward and slightly bent at the elbows.
10. Their fingers should gently rest against you and lightly touch your genitals.
11. Take a few moments to get comfortable.

PAUSE A FEW SECONDS

12. Rock forward and lightly spread powder or oil over your partner's shoulders, neck, and arms, all the way to the fingers.

PAUSE A FEW SECONDS

13. Now gently spread the powder or oil over the area covered using only your fingertips.
14. Start from behind your partner's neck and, using your fingertips only, move down the upper back, shoulders, upper arms, elbows, lower arms, wrists, and fingers.
15. Now work your fingertips back from your partner's fingers back up the hands, forearms, elbows, upper arms, shoulders, upper back, and neck.

PAUSE A FEW SECONDS

16. Now repeat this sequence using the back of your fingernails to gently rake your partner's neck, upper back, shoulders, upper arms, elbows, lower arms, hands, and fingers.
17. Reverse this sequence and use your fingernails to gently rake your partner's fingers, wrists, lower arms, elbows, upper arms, shoulders, upper back, and neck.

PAUSE A FEW SECONDS

18. This time repeat the same sequence, but only after you guide your partner's hands to your genitals so they can feel your penis or vulva as you massage them.

Notice your thoughts, self-talk, mental images, and feelings, as you massage your partner's back.

If your mind wanders into the future or the past or fills with unhelpful thoughts and feelings, note that this is happening and say to yourself, *there goes my runaway mind again, taking me out of the present moment*, and focus on your partner's body and the sensations in your hands and fingers as you massage.

19. Instead of using your fingertips, grasp your partner's skin and muscle with your thumbs and forefingers. Gently roll the muscle in your partner's neck, upper back, shoulders, upper arms, elbows, lower arms, wrists and fingers.

PAUSE A FEW SECONDS

20. Now reverse your motion, using your thumbs and forefingers to massage your partner's fingers, wrists, lower arms, elbows, forearms, shoulders, upper back, and neck.
21. This time, as you move up to your partner's shoulders, rise off of your ankles and hunch over your partner's head.
22. Let your genitals rub up against your partner's hair and head as you finish massaging your partner's neck and shoulders.

PAUSE A FEW SECONDS

Notice your thoughts, self-talk, mental images, and feelings, as you massage your partner's back.

If your mind wanders into the future or the past or fills with unhelpful thoughts and feelings, note that this is happening and say to yourself; *there goes my runaway mind again, taking me out of the present moment*, and focus on your partner's body and the sensations in your hands and fingers as you massage.

23. Now shift your attention to your partner's back, starting at the base of the skull and working down all the way to the crack of your partner's buttocks.
24. Spread powder or oil over this area.
25. Use the light fingertip motion to spread the powder or oil from your partner's neck all the way to your partner's buttocks.
26. Focus on the center of your partner's back a few inches on either side of the spine.

27. Rise off of your ankles and move your body over your partner to reach all the way down to their buttocks.
28. Spread some powder or oil in the crack of your partner's buttocks and gently spread it around with your fingertips.

PAUSE A FEW SECONDS

29. Move back up from your partner's buttocks to the base of your partner's neck, using one continuous motion with the backs of your fingers.
30. Now do one more down and back sequence using your finger tips and the backs of your fingers.

PAUSE A FEW SECONDS

31. Now spread your hands with your fingers pointing away from your partner's spine.
32. Position your hands so that the heels of your hands are about 3 inches away from your partner's spine.
33. Rise up off your heels and lean over your partner, putting your weight on your hands.
34. Press your partner's back from just below the neck all the way to the crack of the buttocks.
35. At the end of your motion you should feel the curve of your partner's spine as you massage over it.
36. Ask your partner about the amount of pressure you are applying and adjust it accordingly.

PAUSE A FEW SECONDS

37. As you return to your kneeling position, move your hands and pull them up along the sides of your partner's buttocks, waist, ribs, chest, and up to the arm pits.

PAUSE A FEW SECONDS

38. Repeat that sequence a couple of times, pressing on the way down and pulling on the way back along the sides.

PAUSE A FEW SECONDS

Notice your thoughts, self-talk, mental images, and feelings, as you massage your partner's back.

If your mind wanders into the future or the past or fills with unhelpful thoughts and feelings note that this is happening and say to yourself, *there goes my runaway mind again, taking me out of the present moment*, and focus on your partner's body and the sensations in your hands and fingers as you massage.

39. Now use your thumbs and entire hands to knead your partner's back muscles as you start from the upper back, work your way down the middle, and end up at your partner's buttocks.
40. Divide your partner's back into four or five sections and stop at each and knead for a few moments before moving lower and lower.

PAUSE A FEW SECONDS

41. Now get up off of the bed and have your partner scooch down so they can fully extend their arms overhead with their elbows slightly bent.
42. Take time to nuzzle your partner's back and buttocks.

PAUSE A FEW SECONDS

43. Get back on the bed and straddle your partner from behind.

DO NOT DO THIS IF YOUR PARTNER HAS ANY BACK PROBLEMS. PROCEED TO STEP 48 AND KNEEL NEXT TO YOUR PARTNER RATHER THAN STRADDLING YOUR PARTNER'S BACK.

44. Your penis or vulva should rest directly over the topmost part of the crack in your partner's buttocks.

PAUSE A FEW SECONDS

45. Use more oil to lubricate the area and let your penis or vulva nestle into the crack of your partner's buttocks.

PAUSE A FEW SECONDS

Notice your thoughts, self-talk, mental images, and feelings, as you massage your partner's back.

If your mind wanders into the future or the past or fills with unhelpful thoughts and feelings, note that this is happening and say to yourself, *there goes my runaway mind again, taking me out of the present moment*, and focus on your partner's body and the sensations in your hands and fingers as you massage.

46. Take the weight off of your partner's body by lifting yourself as you move forward and massage your partner's back from the buttocks up to the neck.
47. Start with light fingertip motions moving up and back from the buttocks to the neck and back.
48. Do this a couple of times.

PAUSE A FEW SECONDS

49. Position your hands so that the heels of your hands are about three inches away from your partner's spine.

50. Rise up off your heels and lean over your partner putting your weight on your hands.
51. Press your partner's back from just above the buttocks all the way to just below the neck.
52. Now move your hands to the sides of your partner's torso and pull your hands back along the sides of your partner's body down to the hips.

PAUSE A FEW SECONDS

53. Repeat this motion again, but this time intentionally slide your genitals back and forth along your partner's buttocks as you move up and down your partner's back.
54. Ask your partner how this pressure feels and adjust it or stop it accordingly.

PAUSE A FEW SECONDS

Notice your thoughts, self-talk, mental images, and feelings, as you massage your partner's back.

If your mind wanders into the future or the past or fills with unhelpful thoughts and feelings, note that this is happening and say to yourself, *there goes my runaway mind again, taking me out of the present moment*, and focus on your partner's body and the sensations in your hands and fingers as you massage.

55. Continue to massage your partner's back and arms, but this time as you press your hands up your partner's back, go all the way up both arms to your partner's fingers.
56. Allow yourself to gently press flat against your partner for a pause before returning back and pulling your hands down along your partner's arms and down the sides of their back.
57. Now close your eyes and examine your partner's neck, head, hair, and shoulders using your senses of touch, smell, and taste.

58. Use your nose, cheeks, face, head, and hair to examine your partner's neck, head, hair, and shoulders.

PAUSE A FEW SECONDS

59. Now take a quick taste. Suck or any part of your partner's neck, shoulders, or back. You don't have to get too freaky—just take a taste

PAUSE A FEW SECONDS

Notice your thoughts, self-talk, mental images and emotions about experiencing your partner's neck, head, hair, and shoulders with all five of your senses.

If your mind wanders into the future or the past or fills with unhelpful thoughts and feelings, note that this is happening and say to yourself, *there goes my runaway mind again, taking me out of the present moment*, and focus on your partner's back.

60. Continue to massage your partner's back for a few more moments, using any strokes you wish.
61. When you are done, gently roll off of your partner and rest side-by-side for a few moments.
62. Use a towel to wipe off the excess oil or powder from your partner and cover them with the towel or blanket.
63. Relax, you have nowhere to go and nothing to do but enjoy this moment.
64. Sometimes giving a back massage is very arousing and is a natural prelude for intercourse.

CHAPTER 15

Mindful Masturbation

Masturbation evolves out of a natural sensual exploration of your own body. As a child you notice that it feels good when you intentionally rub your genitals, or they unintentionally rub up against something. The expression of healthy sexual relationships in adulthood begins with self-exploration from the time of birth. For most of us, masturbation provides our first source of sexual pleasure. It can be a lifelong source of sexual pleasure if your mind allows you to engage in it. To many people, however, masturbation is associated with juvenile, sinful, or inappropriate sexual behavior.

Centuries upon centuries of misinformation based on religious teaching and pseudoscience have clouded the truth about masturbation and have shrouded the topic in a veil of sin, shame, guilt, and punishment. In reality, masturbation is not a juvenile behavior, does not cause any physical problems and carries no risk for any physical or psychological illness. Contrary to popular belief, you cannot masturbate to excess. It is a self-limiting behavior; you will ultimately lose your interest in it and start doing something else. As long as you follow basic hygienic precautions (clean hands, toys, and so on) and have adequate lubrication, you can masturbate as often as you want to. Rather than being viewed as a problem, masturbation can be looked at as a healthy outlet for sexual desire. It can reduce your risk for sexually transmitted diseases if you don't have a safe sexual partner, and is an alternative to having sex with prostitutes or anonymous partners.

Masturbating on a regular basis may even decrease your risk for developing prostate cancer. In a study of over 2,000 men between the ages of 20-50, Giles et al. (2003) found that the more often they ejaculated through masturbation, the less likely they were to develop prostate cancer. The prostate gland produces fluid that contributes to the make-up of semen and ejaculation cleanses the prostate and prevents carcinogens from building up. Men who masturbated to ejaculation on a regular basis had a lower incidence of prostate cancer than men who climaxed through partnered activity.

Autoeroticism

Autoeroticism is the catch-all term used to describe sexual desire or gratification experienced by a person without the direct participation of a partner. Autoeroticism is fueled by sexual fantasy and is usually accompanied by masturbation.

There are many forms of sexual stimuli used in autoerotic activities. These include, but are not limited to, adult books and magazines, films, CD-ROMs, videos, telephone sex, cybersex via computer webcams, chat rooms, and video clips. Most autoerotic stimuli revolve around fairly standardized sexual fantasies, but are limited only by your imagination. The most common themes portrayed in autoerotic material include sex with a stranger, sex with a same sex partner, group sex, sex in embarrassing places/situations, receiving or giving oral sex, forced sex, or spontaneous sex with a stranger at home, work, or other places (Blonna and Carter, 2018).

An interesting finding from one of the most extensive studies of autoerotic behavior showed that contrary to popular belief, autoerotic activity was not limited to people who did not have sexual partners and viewed it as a less desirable form of sexual behavior. Instead, they found that people with higher levels of partnered sex engaged in higher levels of autoerotic sex. Rather than using autoerotic activities to compensate for the lack of a sex partner, they used them as a source of additional sexual pleasure in the relationship. In addition, the study found that those with higher levels of autoerotic activity were more likely than those with lower levels to engage in a broader range of sexual activities (Lauman et al, 1994). This might have to do with them having a more elaborate set of personal sexual scripts that allowed them to try different things with their partners.

Sexual Fantasy

You might ask, "What exactly is a sexual fantasy?" For the purpose of this book and understanding ACT better, think of sexual fantasies as a category of personal scripts and mental images. The main difference between your sexual fantasies and your other personal scripts and mental images, however, is that they have the ability to turn you on. Your sexual fantasies can fuel your sexual desire and trigger your sexual response. In that respect, they are very different from all other categories of personal scripts and mental images, and therefore, important to discuss.

Sexual fantasies serve many important functions. Fantasies help you expand your sexual repertoire and develop new personal scripts. In your fantasies you can play with new sexual behaviors and lifestyles from the safety of your own mind. Coupled with masturbation, they provide a safe, exciting venue for the release of your sexual tension. Your sexual fantasies provide a "practice arena" to work through sexual scripts and encounters that you may, or may not, want to enact in real life. This safe practice carries none of the interpersonal or health risks associated with actually having sex with another person.

Mindful Masturbation Exercise # 1: Mindful Masturbation (for her)

Purpose: Couples sometimes get stuck in a sexual rut because they shift their focus off of the couple and onto the individual. *He* feels angry because his needs are not being met or *she* feels angry because she isn't getting enough sexual attention. This activity shifts the focus off of the self and onto the partner. It also introduces masturbation into the relationship in a very non-threatening way. Masturbating your partner is a selfless act that can substitute for intercourse on those occasions where one partner is not in the mood for intercourse but still wants to please the other.

The following is a set of preliminary instructions to use for all of the mindful sex activities.

1. Make sure to read all of the instructions for this exercise before doing it with your partner.
2. This will ensure that there are no surprises and you are comfortable with the instructions.
3. Allow 30 minutes of uninterrupted time for each activity.
4. Do this and all of the other mindful sex activities in the bedroom on your own bed.
5. Make sure the room is at a temperature that you and your partner find relaxing.
6. Put relaxing background music on that will help cancel out distracting sounds from the outside environment.
7. Make sure that the music you choose is instrumental and has no singing. Songs tend to distract your mind and take the focus off of the activity and onto thinking about the music.
8. Turn off your cell phone, television, and any distracting device.
9. Burn your favorite scented candle or incense.
10. Take a shower or bath with your partner before engaging in any of these activities.
11. Be mindful of the warmth of the water, the smell and feel of your partner and the soap as you move it over your partner's body and get clean and ready for these mindful sex activities.
12. When performing this activity keep your mind on your partner's body. Focus your attention on what each motion feels like and how your partner responds to your actions.

13. When your mind drifts to the past or future, or starts "thinking" or "worrying" about if you are doings things right or perfect, just get back to noticing, without judgment, what each motion feels like and how your partner responds to your actions.
14. Whenever your mind drifts, say to yourself, *there goes my runaway mind again taking me out of the present moment*, and shift your focus back on what you are doing to your partner.

That's it for general instructions. I will talk you through each activity, step by step.

Relax and enjoy the process.

Specific Instructions

Before following these instructions, make sure that you have read and followed the preliminary instructions.

1. Lie down next to your partner on the bed so you can face her as you masturbate her with your hand.
2. Spend a few moments just noticing your partner's vulva.
3. Get close and examine her pubic area, vaginal lips, perineum (the area between her vaginal and anal openings.)
4. Carefully part her vaginal lips and examine her clitoris.
5. Imagine that you are a scientist taking notes about the size, shape, color, and texture of your partner's vulva.

PAUSE A FEW SECONDS

6. Now close your eyes and examine your partner's vulva using your senses of touch, smell, and taste.
7. Use your nose, cheeks, face, head, and hair to examine your partner's vulva.

PAUSE A FEW SECONDS

8. Now take a quick taste. You just washed your partner's vulva so it is clean. Suck or lick any part of your partner's vulva. Don't start having oral sex, just take a taste.

PAUSE A FEW SECONDS

Notice your thoughts, self-talk, mental images and emotions about experiencing your partner's vulva with all five of your senses.

If your mind wanders into the future or the past or fills with unhelpful thoughts and feelings note that this is happening and say to yourself, *there goes my runaway mind again, taking me out of the present moment*, and focus on your partner's vulva.

9. Put some oil, lotion, or jelly on your partner's pubic area above her vagina.
10. Lightly swirl the lubrication around her entire pubic area with your fingertips only.

PAUSE A FEW SECONDS

11. Continue spreading the lubricant, but this time stroke the area using the front and back of your fingertips as you move up and down.

PAUSE A FEW SECONDS

12. Focus your attention on the sensations emanating from her pubic area and your fingertips.

PAUSE A FEW SECONDS

Continue to stroke your partner and notice your thoughts, self-talk, mental images, and feelings, as you stroke your partner's pubic area.

If your mind wanders into the future or the past or fills with unhelpful thoughts and feelings, note that this is happening and say to yourself, *there goes my runaway mind again, taking me out of the present moment*, and focus on your partner's body and the sensations in your hands and fingers as you stroke your partner.

13. Now shift back to massaging your partner's pubic area using your fingertips in a circular motion.
14. Continue to massage your partner's pubic area for a few moments.

PAUSE A FEW SECONDS

15. Now increase the pressure on your partner's pubic area by using your entire hand— the fingers, palm, and heel of your hand—to massage the area.
16. Ask your partner how much pressure and motion she desires.
17. Do not put any direct pressure on your partner's clitoris yet.

PAUSE A FEW SECONDS

18. Experiment with different levels of pressure and types of motion, but keep the stimulation limited to the pubic area.
19. Focus your attention on the sensations emanating from your partner's pubic area and your hand and fingers.

Continue to massage your partner's pubic area as you notice your thoughts, self-talk, mental images, and feelings.

If your mind wanders into the future or the past or fills with unhelpful thoughts and feelings, note that this is happening and say to yourself, *there goes my runaway mind again, taking me out of the present moment*, and focus on your partner's body and the sensations in your hands and fingers as you massage your partner's pubic area.

PAUSE A FEW SECONDS

20. Now shift your attention to your partner's vaginal lips—the folds of skin that protect the opening of her vagina.
21. Notice that the very top of her lips form a fold that covers her clitoris.
22. Gently part this fold and notice your partner's clitoris and the opening to her vagina.
23. Put some oil, lotion, or jelly on your partner's vaginal lips, using your thumb and fingertips.
24. Lightly roll each vaginal lip with your thumb and forefinger, moving up and down the entire length of her vaginal lips.
25. Take your time. You have nowhere to go and nothing to do but massage your partner's vaginal lips.

PAUSE A FEW SECONDS

26. Now switch to a stroking motion and use your fingertips and the back of your fingertips and knuckles to massage your partner's vaginal lips.
27. Do not touch her clitoris directly when doing this. Part your fingers when working up and down to go around her clitoris.

PAUSE A FEW SECONDS

28. Continue to massage your partner's vaginal lips, but now gently tug them back and forth and up and down, indirectly stimulating her clitoris this way.

PAUSE A FEW SECONDS

Continue to massage your partner's vaginal lips as you notice your thoughts, self-talk, mental images, and feelings.

If your mind wanders into the future or the past or fills with unhelpful thoughts and feelings, note that this is happening and say to yourself, *there goes my runaway mind again, taking me out of the present moment,* and focus on your partner's body and the sensations in your hands and fingers as you massage your partner's vaginal lips.

PAUSE A FEW SECONDS

29. Now shift your attention to your partner's clitoris and gently massage it using your fingertips.
30. Use a swirling motion to move her clitoris around and around.
31. Try experimenting with varying amounts of direct pressure on the head of your partner's clitoris.
32. Ask your partner if you are using the right pressure and swirling motion.

PAUSE A FEW SECONDS

33. Continue to stimulate your partner's clitoris, but this time use your thumb and forefinger to grasp it and swirl it.
34. Gently tug her clitoris as you swirl it.
35. Now try stimulating your partner's clitoris by using indirect pressure on it, by massaging the topmost fold of her vaginal lips where they meet at her clitoris.
36. Ask your partner if you are using the right pressure and tugging motion.

PAUSE A FEW SECONDS

As you continue to stimulate your partner's clitoris, notice your thoughts, self-talk, mental images, and feelings, as you massage it.

If your mind wanders into the future or the past or fills with unhelpful thoughts and feelings, note that this is happening and say to yourself, *there goes my runaway mind again, taking me out of the present moment,* and focus on your partner's body and the sensations in your thumb and finger as you stimulate your partner's clitoris.

37. Put some oil, lotion, or jelly on your partner's perineum, the area between her vaginal and anal openings.
38. Lightly swirl the lubrication around your partner's perineum with your fingertips only.
39. Try experimenting with varying amounts of pressure and motion on your partner's perineum.
40. Ask your partner which level of pressure and type of motion feels the best.

PAUSE A FEW SECONDS

41. Now shift your attention to your partner's entire vulva and vaginal opening.
42. Spend a few moments just noticing this area.
43. Get close and examine her pubic area, vaginal lips, clitoris, and perineum now that she is aroused.
44. Notice the changes in the size, shape, and color of her vaginal lips and clitoris.

PAUSE A FEW SECONDS

45. Now gently insert one well-lubricated finger into your partner's vagina and move it in a slow circular motion.
46. Focus your attention on the sensations emanating from your partner's vagina and your finger as you gently move it in a circular motion.

PAUSE A FEW SECONDS

47. Experiment with the depth of your finger and pace of your motion as you move your finger in a circular motion in your partner's vagina.
48. If your partner is comfortable with you inserting more than one finger into her vagina, experiment with inserting more than one finger into her vagina and moving them in a circular motion.

PAUSE A FEW SECONDS

49. Now combine the circular motion of your finger or fingers with pressure on your partner's clitoris using the heel of your hand. You might find that stimulating her clitoris with the fingers or heel of your opposite hands works better for you in providing clitoral stimulation.

PAUSE A FEW SECONDS

Continue to stimulate your partner's vagina and clitoris and notice your thoughts, self-talk, mental images, and feelings, as you do this.

If your mind wanders into the future or the past or fills with unhelpful thoughts and feelings, note that this is happening and say to yourself, *there goes my runaway mind again, taking me out of the present moment*, and focus on your partner's body and the sensations in your hands and fingers as you stimulate your partner's vagina and clitoris.

PAUSE A FEW SECONDS

50. Now switch from a circular motion to an in and out thrusting.
51. Thrust your finger or fingers in and out of your partner's vagina.
52. Experiment with the depth and pace of your thrusting.
53. Ask your partner what type of thrusting she desires.

PAUSE A FEW SECONDS

54. Now combine thrusting in and out with applying pressure on your partner's clitoris using the heel of your hand.
55. You might find that stimulating her clitoris with the fingers or heel of your opposite hands works better for you in providing clitoral stimulation.

56. Continue masturbating your partner with any of the types of stimulation, pressure, and, pace that are pleasurable for her.

PAUSE A FEW SECONDS

57. Continue with them until she reaches an orgasm or asks you to stop.
58. After your partner has her orgasm or asks you to stop, lie quietly and pay attention to the sensations in your and your partner's bodies.
59. Allow your partner's body to relax, her vaginal area to return to a non-aroused state, and her breathing to return to normal before getting up.
60. Relax. You have nothing to do and nowhere to go for the next few minutes.

Notice your thoughts, self-talk, mental images, and feelings, as you massage your partner's back.

If your mind wanders into the future or the past or fills with unhelpful thoughts and feelings, note that this is happening and say to yourself, *there goes my runaway mind again, taking me out of the present moment*, and focus on your partner's body and the sensations of lying next to her.

Mindful Masturbation Exercise # 2: Mindful Masturbation (for him)

Purpose: Couples sometimes get stuck in a sexual rut because they shift their focus off of the couple and onto the individual. *He* feels angry because his needs are not being met or *she* feels angry because she isn't getting enough sexual attention. This activity shifts the focus off of the self and onto the partner. It also introduces masturbation into the relationship in a very non-threatening way. Masturbating your partner is a selfless act that can substitute for intercourse on those occasions where one partner is not in the mood for intercourse but still wants to please the other.

The following is a set of preliminary instructions to use for all of the mindful sex activities.

1. Read the complete set of instructions for whatever mindful sex exercise you choose to engage in before doing it with your partner.
2. This will ensure that there are no surprises and you are comfortable with the instructions.
3. Allow 30 minutes of uninterrupted time for each activity.
4. Do this and all of the other mindful sex activities in the bedroom on your own bed.
5. Make sure the room is at a temperature that you and your partner find relaxing.
6. Put relaxing background music on that will help cancel out distracting sounds from the outside environment.
7. Make sure that the music you choose is instrumental and has no singing. Songs tend to distract your mind and take the focus off of the activity and onto thinking about the music.
8. Turn off your cell phone, television, and any distracting device.
9. Burn your favorite scented candle or incense.
10. Take a shower or bath with your partner before engaging in any of these activities.
11. Be mindful of the warmth of the water, the smell and feel of your partner and the soap as you move it over your partner's body and get clean and ready for these mindful sex activities.
12. When performing this activity keep your mind on your partner's body. Focus your attention on what each motion feels like and how your partner responds to your actions.
13. When your mind drifts to the past or future, or starts "thinking" or "worrying" about if you are doings things right or perfect, just get back to noticing, without judgment, what each motion feels like and how your partner responds to your actions.

14. Whenever your mind drifts, say to yourself, *there goes my runaway mind again taking me out of the present moment*, and shift your focus back on what you are doing to your partner.

That's it for general instructions. I will talk you through each activity, step by step. Relax and enjoy the process.

Specific Instructions

Before following these instructions, make sure that you have read and followed the preliminary instructions.

1. Lie down next to your partner on the bed so you can face him as you masturbate him with your hand.
2. Spend a few moments just noticing your partner's penis and scrotum.
3. Get close and examine his penis, testicles and scrotum, and his perineum (the area between his scrotum and anal opening.)
4. Imagine that you are a scientist taking notes about the size, shape, color, and texture of your partner's genitals.

PAUSE A FEW SECONDS

5. Now close your eyes and examine your partner's genitals using your senses of touch, smell, and taste.
6. Use your nose, cheeks, face, head, and hair to examine your partner's penis, scrotum, and entire genital area.

PAUSE A FEW SECONDS

7. Now take a quick taste. You just washed your partner's genitals so they are clean. Suck or lick any part of your partner's genitals. Don't start having oral sex—just take a taste.

PAUSE A FEW SECONDS

Notice your thoughts, self-talk, mental images and emotions about experiencing your partner's genitals with all five of your senses.

Whenever your mind drifts, say to yourself, *there goes my runaway mind again, taking me out of the present moment*, and focus on your partner's genitals.

8. Put some oil, lotion, or jelly on the head of your partner's penis.
9. Lightly swirl the lubrication around the head of your partner's penis with your fingertips only.

PAUSE A FEW SECONDS

10. Focus your attention on the sensations emanating from the tip of your partner's penis and your fingertips.

Note the thoughts, feelings, self-talk, and mental images that accompany your actions.

If your mind wanders into the future or the past or fills with unhelpful thoughts and feelings, note that this is happening and say to yourself, *there goes my runaway mind again, taking me out of the present moment*, and focus on your partner's body and the sensations in your hands and fingers as you masturbate your partner.

PAUSE A FEW SECONDS

11. Now use your thumb and middle two fingers to swirl the lubrication around the head of your partner's penis.
12. Use your three fingers to apply pressure to your circular motion. Experiment with different levels of pressure, but keep the stimulation limited to just the head of your partner's penis.
13. Ask your partner what kind of pressure he likes and adjust your pressure accordingly.

PAUSE A FEW SECONDS

14. Now shift your attention to the shaft of your partner's penis, the area that extends from the head to his testicles (balls).
15. Put some oil, lotion, or jelly on the shaft of your partner's penis and your fingertips.
16. Lightly move your fingers up and down and around the shaft of your partner's penis with your fingertips only. Do not grab hold of his penis, just stroke it gently with your fingertips.

PAUSE A FEW SECONDS

17. Focus your attention on the sensations emanating from the shaft of your partner's penis and your fingertips.

Note the thoughts, feelings, self-talk, and mental images that accompany your actions.

If your mind wanders into the future or the past or fills with unhelpful thoughts and feelings, note that this is happening and say to yourself, *there goes my runaway mind again, taking me out of the present moment*, and focus on your partner's body and the sensations in your hands and fingers as you masturbate your partner.

PAUSE A FEW SECONDS

18. Now wrap your hand around the shaft of your partner's penis and apply pressure as you stroke his penis with your hand. Experiment with different levels of pressure and the speed of your stroking motion.
19. Ask your partner what kind of pressure and speed he likes and adjust your stroking motion accordingly.

PAUSE A FEW SECONDS

20. Put some oil, lotion, or jelly on your partner's testicles.

21. Lightly swirl the lubrication around your partner's testicles with your fingertips only.

PAUSE A FEW SECONDS

22. Focus your attention on the sensations emanating from your partner's testicles, penis, and your fingertips.

Note the thoughts, feelings, self-talk, and mental images that accompany your actions.

If your mind wanders into the future or the past or fills with unhelpful thoughts and feelings, note that this is happening and say to yourself, *there goes my runaway mind again, taking me out of the present moment*, and focus on your partner's body and the sensations in your hands and fingers as you masturbate your partner.

PAUSE A FEW SECONDS

23. Now wrap your hand around your partner's testicles and apply pressure as you knead his testicles using your hand. Experiment with different levels of pressure and the speed of your kneading motion.
24. Be careful and start very gently, as this is a very sensitive area.
25. Ask your partner what kind of pressure and speed he likes and adjust your stroking motion accordingly.
26. Continue this motion for a few moments.

PAUSE A FEW SECONDS

27. Now shift your attention to your partner's entire genital area.
28. Spend a few moments just noticing this area.
29. Get close and examine his penis, testicles, scrotum, and perineum, now that he is aroused.

30. Notice the changes in the size, shape, and color of his penis, testicles, and scrotum.

Note the thoughts, feelings, self-talk, and mental images that accompany your actions as you examine your partner's genitals.

If your mind wanders into the future or the past or fills with unhelpful thoughts and feelings, note that this is happening and say to yourself, *there goes my runaway mind again, taking me out of the present moment*, and focus on your partner's genitals.

PAUSE A FEW SECONDS

31. Now put some oil, lotion, or jelly on your partner's perineum (the area between his testicles and his anal opening).
32. Lightly swirl the lubrication around your partner's perineum with your fingertips only.

PAUSE A FEW SECONDS

33. Focus your attention on the sensations emanating from your partner's entire penis, testicles, perineum, and your hand.

PAUSE A FEW SECONDS

34. Now go back and wrap your hand around the shaft of your partner's penis, apply pressure, and then increase the pressure and speed of your stroking and other motions.
35. Ask him what pressure, speed, and motions he needs in order to climax.

Note the thoughts, feelings, self-talk, and mental images that accompany your actions as you get ready to make your partner come.

If your mind wanders into the future or the past or fills with unhelpful thoughts and feelings, note that this is happening and say to yourself, *there goes my runaway mind again, taking me out of the present moment,* and focus on your partner's body and the sensations in your hands and fingers as you masturbate him.

36. Continue your stroking and other motions until your partner climaxes.
37. After your partner ejaculates, lie quietly and pay attention to the sensations in his genital area and the rest of his body as he winds down.
38. Let his penis go limp and his breathing return to normal before getting up and washing him off with a warm wash cloth and dry towel.
39. Relax. You have nothing to do and nowhere to go for the next few minutes.

Note the thoughts, feelings, self-talk, and mental images that accompany your actions as you get ready to make your partner come.

If your mind wanders into the future or the past or fills with unhelpful thoughts and feelings, note that this is happening and say to yourself, *there goes my runaway mind again, taking me out of the present moment*, and focus on your partner's body and the sensations in your body as you lie down next to him.

CHAPTER 16

Mindful Oral Sex

Oral sex is the stimulation of your partner's genitals with your lips, mouth, tongue, and face. The three main types of oral sex are fellatio (mouth-to-penis contact), cunnilingus (mouth-to-vulva contact), and analingus (mouth-to-anus contact). All three are common forms of sexual expression for straight, gay, lesbian, and bisexual people.

Fellatio, also known as a "blow job," involves licking and sucking a man's penis. Many men find that a combination of oral and manual stimulation of the penis is necessary to provide enough stimulation for orgasm. Since orgasm in men is accompanied by ejaculation, couples need to discuss their thoughts and feelings about this. If the partner finds swallowing ejaculate distasteful, an alternative is fellatio to the point of orgasm, then withdrawing the penis and ejaculating outside the partner's mouth, or switching to some other form of sexual behavior prior to the point of orgasm.

The oral stimulation of a woman's vulva through licking, sucking, and nibbling or rubbing with the face is called cunnilingus. Although cunnilingus by definition refers to oral stimulation of the vulva, often the perineum and outer parts of the vagina are also stimulated during this act. As with fellatio, cunnilingus can be performed with or without manual stimulation. Many women derive pleasure from having their partner insert a well lubricated finger into their vagina or anus while performing cunnilingus. Saliva or vaginal lubrication can be used to make the fingers slippery. The partner also can stimulate the woman's clitoris with manual stimulation while licking or sucking on another part of the vulva.

Mutual oral sex is often referred to as sixty-nine because of the shape couples form when engaged in it. Mutual oral sex is accomplished in the side-to-side starting point, with each partner's head at the other's genitals. From this position, both partners have easy access to their partner's genitals. From the side-to-side starting point, it is easy to roll into the man or woman on either the top or bottom positions. By being on the top or the bottom, a person can control for deeper penetration of the tongue when performing cunnilingus, or the penis during fellatio. Mutual oral sex is enjoyed by heterosexual, gay, and lesbian couples.

Although it isn't as common as fellatio or cunnilingus, analingus, also known as rimming, is another form of oral sex practiced by people of all forms of sexual orientation. During analingus, a person kisses, licks, or sucks his or her partner's anus. The motions and activities of analingus are similar to both cunnilingus and fellatio. Performing analingus affords a good opportunity to stimulate the perineum, an area richly endowed with nerve endings. Some men and women enjoy having their partners insert their tongue into their anus during analingus. Others prefer that their partner insert a well-lubricated finger into the rectum.

When performing analingus on a woman, care must be taken to avoid spreading Escherichia coli bacteria into the vagina. The tongue or fingers never should be inserted directly from the anus to the vagina without first being washed. Another concern is the spread of hepatitis and other STD organisms through analingus. Because of this, it is not recommended that you perform analingus with a casual sex partner or someone whose STD status is unknown, as this could result in ingesting disease-causing organisms.

Mindful Oral Sex Exercise # 1: Mindful Oral Sex (for him)

Purpose: Couples sometimes get stuck in a sexual rut because they shift their focus off of the couple and onto the individual. *He* feels angry because his needs are not being met or *she* feels angry because she isn't getting enough sexual attention. This activity shifts the focus off of the self and onto the partner. It also introduces oral sex into the relationship in a very nonthreatening way. Going down on your partner is a selfless act that can substitute for intercourse on those occasions where one partner is not in the mood for intercourse but still wants to please the other.

The following is a set of preliminary instructions to use for all of the mindful sex activities.

1. Read the full instructions for whatever mindful sex activity you choose to engage in before doing it with your partner.
2. This will ensure that there are no surprises and you are comfortable with the instructions.
3. Allow 30 minutes of uninterrupted time for each activity.
4. Do this and all of the other mindful sex activities in the bedroom on your own bed.
5. Make sure the room is at a temperature that you and your partner find relaxing.
6. Put relaxing background music on that will help cancel out distracting sounds from the outside environment.
7. Make sure that the music you choose is instrumental and has no singing. Songs tend to distract your mind and take the focus off of the activity and onto thinking about the music.
8. Turn off your cell phone, television, and any distracting device.
9. Burn your favorite scented candle or incense.
10. Take a shower or bath with your partner before engaging in any of these activities.
11. Be mindful of the warmth of the water, the smell and feel of your partner and the soap as you move it over your partner's body and get clean and ready for these mindful sex activities.
12. When performing this activity, keep your mind on your partner's body. Focus your attention on what each motion feels like and how your partner responds to your actions.

13. When your mind drifts to the past or future, or starts "thinking" or "worrying" about if you are doings things right or perfect, just get back to noticing, without judgment, what each motion feels like and how your partner responds to your actions.
14. Whenever your mind drifts, say to yourself, *there goes my runaway mind again, taking me out of the present moment*, and shift your focus back on what you are doing to your partner.

That's it for general instructions. I will talk you through each activity, step by step. Relax and enjoy the process.

Specific Instructions

Before following these instructions, make sure that you have read and completed the preliminary instructions.

1. Lie down next to your partner on the bed so you can face him as you give him oral sex.
2. Spend a few moments just noticing your partner's penis and scrotum.
3. Get close and examine his penis, testicles and scrotum, and his perineum (the area between his scrotum and anal opening.)
4. Imagine that you are a scientist taking notes about the size, shape, color, and texture of your partner's genitals.

PAUSE A FEW SECONDS

5. Now close your eyes and examine your partner's genitals using your senses of touch, smell, and taste.
6. Use your nose, cheeks, face, head, and hair to examine your partner's penis, scrotum, and entire genital area. If he is uncircumcised gently retract his foreskin and continue your exploration and the rest of the activity with his foreskin retracted.

PAUSE A FEW SECONDS

7. Now take a quick taste. You just washed your partner's genitals so they are clean. Suck or lick any part of your partner's genitals. Don't start having oral sex—just take a taste.

Notice your thoughts, self-talk, mental images and emotions about experiencing your partner's genitals with all five of your senses.

If your mind wanders into the future or the past or fills with unhelpful thoughts and feelings note that this is happening and say to yourself, there goes my runaway mind again, taking me out of the present moment, and focus on your partner's genitals.

8. Lightly swirl around your fingertips and the back of your fingers around your partner's penis, scrotum, and entire pubic area.

PAUSE A FEW SECONDS

9. Gently rake your fingernails over the same area.

PAUSE A FEW SECONDS

10. Notice the effects of your fingers on your partner.

PAUSE A FEW SECONDS

11. Continue to do this for a little while.

PAUSE A FEW SECONDS

12. Relax. You have nowhere to go and nothing to do except please your partner.

PAUSE A FEW SECONDS

13. Now get comfortable kneeling or lying next to your partner so you can easily take your partner's penis into your mouth.

14. Take a few seconds to find your most comfortable position.

PAUSE A FEW SECONDS

15. Gently lick your partner's penis, scrotum, and entire pubic area for a few moments.

PAUSE A FEW SECONDS

16. Notice the effects of your movements on your partner's penis, scrotum, and the rest of his body.

PAUSE A FEW SECONDS

17. Now take your partner's penis into your mouth. If he is erect, you can control how much of his penis you take by holding it in your hand. This will keep you from gagging by accidentally taking in more than is comfortable.

PAUSE A FEW SECONDS

18. Gently suck on your partner's penis as you move your head back and forth to create an in and out motion. This simulates him thrusting his penis in and out of you.

PAUSE A FEW SECONDS

Notice your thoughts, self-talk, mental images and emotions as you begin to lick and suck on your partner's penis.

If your mind wanders into the future or the past or fills with unhelpful thoughts and feelings, note that this is happening and say to yourself, *there goes my runaway mind again, taking me out of the present moment*, and focus on your partner's penis.

19. After a few moments of doing this, change actions and go back to licking your partner's penis. This will give your mouth and neck a rest from the sucking and back and forth motion.

PAUSE A FEW SECONDS

20. Take your time and notice the size, shape, and color of the head of his penis as you use your tongue to lick and swirl around it.

PAUSE A FEW SECONDS

21. Move your attention to the underside of his penis. Notice the size, shape, texture, and taste of his penis as you lick the underside all the way up to the tip.

PAUSE A FEW SECONDS

22. The underside, where the shaft meets the head of his penis, contains the most nerve endings of his entire penis so spend time coming back to this area. He will really love this.

PAUSE A FEW SECONDS

23. Now take your partner's penis back into your mouth. Try to take a little more of it in than you did at first.
24. Remember, you can control how much of his penis you take by holding it in your hand. This will keep you from gagging by accidentally taking in more than is comfortable.
25. Don't worry about being able to take all of it into your mouth and down to your throat.
26. While this is a common theme in pornography, not everyone is comfortable taking their partner's entire penis deep into their throat.
27. Relax and enjoy what you are doing rather than thinking about what you "should" be doing.

PAUSE A FEW SECONDS

28. Continue to suck on your partner's penis as you move your head back and forth to create an in and out motion.
29. Use your tongue to swirl around his penis, particularly the head, as you move your head back and forth.

PAUSE A FEW SECONDS

30. Use your hand to pump your partner's penis as you suck on it and swirl your tongue.
31. Vary the pressure and speed of your pumping as you swirl your tongue around the head of his penis.
32. If your partner begins to thrust his penis in and out of your mouth it is up to you to either allow this, control the depth of the thrust with your hand, or ask him to stop.
33. If you do not want him to do this, simply take his penis out of your mouth and say, "Not now, I prefer to control the thrusting."
34. Return to sucking, licking, and pumping your partner's penis with your hand as you move your head back and forth.

PAUSE A FEW SECONDS

Notice your thoughts, self-talk, mental images and emotions as you lick, suck, and pump your partner's penis.

If your mind wanders into the future or the past or fills with unhelpful thoughts and feelings, note that this is happening and say to yourself, *there goes my runaway mind again, taking me out of the present moment*, and focus on your partner's penis.

35. Now shift your attention to his scrotum.
36. Notice the size, shape, texture, and taste of his scrotum as you lick it and gently suck on it.

PAUSE A FEW SECONDS

37. GENTLY take each testicle in your mouth and lick and suck on them one at a time. This is a very sensitive area and guys vary tremendously regarding how much pressure they like.
38. Stop and ask your partner, "How is the pressure?" just to double-check.

PAUSE A FEW SECONDS

39. If you are comfortable with it, lick the area between his anal opening and his scrotum. This area is an often overlooked erogenous zone.
40. Spend a few moments licking this area.

PAUSE A FEW SECONDS

41. Now shift your focus back to his penis and use your hand to gently masturbate him as you swirl your tongue around the head of his penis, focusing on the sensitive underside.
42. Spend a few moments doing this.

PAUSE A FEW SECONDS

43. Now put your partner's penis back in your mouth and increase the intensity of your sucking and back and forth head motion.
44. At this point your partner might increase his thrusting as he is probably getting ready to come.
45. Once again, it is up to you to either allow, control, or stop this.
46. Continue to increase the intensity of your sucking and back and forth head motion as you continue this for a few moments.

PAUSE A FEW SECONDS

47. Now take his penis out of your mouth and use your hand to masturbate him. At this point you should be able to sense if your partner is ready to come. His legs will start tensing, his toes will start curling, and other muscles will get tighter and more tense. His breathing will also increase.
48. Notice what is going on in your partner's genitals and the rest of his body as you continue to masturbate him and lick and suck on his penis.

PAUSE A FEW SECONDS

49. If your partner is ready to come you can finish him off with your hand or your mouth.
50. If you finish him with your mouth you can either capture his ejaculation in your mouth and spit it out or swallow it.
51. This is your decision to make. Your partner will enjoy the orgasm however you decide to finish.

Notice your thoughts, self-talk, mental images and emotions as you make your partner come.

If your mind wanders into the future or the past or fills with unhelpful thoughts and feelings, note that this is happening and say to yourself, *there goes my runaway mind again, taking me out of the present moment*, and focus on your partner's orgasm.

52. Relax, and continue with whatever motions you wish until your partner comes.

PAUSE A FEW SECONDS

53. Spend a few moments, squeezing, licking, and sucking your partner's penis immediately after he comes.

54. This is intensely pleasurable, so do not rush this step.

PAUSE A FEW SECONDS

55. If you finished off your partner with your hand or spit his ejaculate onto his belly, take a moment and get a warm wash cloth and towel and clean him off.

PAUSE A FEW SECONDS

56. Now is cuddle time. Curl up with your partner and just relax. You both deserve it.

PAUSE A FEW SECONDS

Mindful Oral Sex Exercise # 2: Mindful Oral Sex (for her)

Purpose: Couples sometimes get stuck in a sexual rut because they shift their focus off of the couple and onto the individual. *He* feels angry because his needs are not being met or *she* feels angry because she isn't getting enough sexual attention. This activity shifts the focus off of the self and onto the partner. It also introduces oral sex into the relationship in a very nonthreatening way. Going down on your partner is a selfless act that can substitute for intercourse on those occasions where one partner is not in the mood for intercourse but still wants to please the other.

The following is a set of preliminary instructions to use for all of the mindful sex activities.

1. Read the full set of instructions for whatever mindful sex activity you choose to engage in before doing it with your partner.

2. This will ensure that there are no surprises and you are comfortable with the instructions.
3. Allow 30 minutes of uninterrupted time for each activity.
4. Do this and all of the other mindful sex activities in the bedroom on your own bed.
5. Make sure the room is at a temperature that you and your partner find relaxing.
6. Put relaxing background music on that will help cancel out distracting sounds from the outside environment..
7. Make sure that the music you choose is instrumental and has no singing. Songs tend to distract your mind and take the focus off of the activity and onto thinking about the music.
8. Turn off your cell phone, television, and any distracting device.
9. Burn your favorite scented candle or incense.
10. Take a shower or bath with your partner before engaging in any of these activities.
11. Be mindful of the warmth of the water, the smell and feel of your partner and the soap as you move it over your partner's body and get clean and ready for these mindful sex activities.
12. When performing this activity keep your mind on your partner's body. Focus your attention on what each motion feels like and how your partner responds to your actions.
13. When your mind drifts to the past or future, or starts "thinking" or "worrying" about if you are doings things right or perfect, just get back to noticing, without judgment, what each motion feels like and how your partner responds to your actions.
14. Whenever your mind drifts, say to yourself, *there goes my runaway mind again taking me out of the present moment*, and shift your focus back on what you are doing to your partner.

That's it for general instructions. I will talk you through each activity, step by step. Relax and enjoy the process.

Specific Instructions

Before following these instructions make sure that you have read and followed the preliminary instructions.

1. Lie down next to your partner on the bed so you can face her as you give her oral sex.
2. Spend a few moments just noticing your partner's vulva.
3. Get close and examine her pubic area, vaginal lips, perineum (the area between her vaginal and anal openings).
4. Carefully part her vaginal lips and examine her clitoris.
5. Imagine that you are a scientist taking notes about the size, shape, color, and texture of your partner's vulva.

PAUSE A FEW SECONDS

6. Now close your eyes and examine your partner's vulva using your senses of touch, smell, and taste.
7. Use your nose, cheeks, face, head, and hair to examine your partner's vulva.

PAUSE A FEW SECONDS

8. Now take a quick taste. You just washed your partner's vulva so it is clean. Suck or lick any part of your partner's vulva and get a taste of what is to come.

Notice your thoughts, self-talk, mental images and emotions about experiencing your partner's vulva with all five of your senses.

If your mind wanders into the future or the past or fills with unhelpful thoughts and feelings, note that this is happening and say to yourself, *there goes my runaway mind again, taking me out of the present moment*, and focus on your partner's vulva.

9. Have your partner lie on her back on your bed.
10. Lightly swirl around your fingertips and the backs of your fingers around your partner's vaginal lips, clitoris, and entire pubic area.

PAUSE A FEW SECONDS

11. Gently rake your fingernails over the same area.

PAUSE A FEW SECONDS

12. Notice the effects of your fingers on your partner.

PAUSE A FEW SECONDS

13. Continue to do this for a little while longer.

PAUSE A FEW SECONDS

14. Relax. You have nowhere to go and nothing to do except please your partner.

PAUSE A FEW SECONDS

15. Now get comfortable kneeling or lying next to your partner so you can easily reach your partner's vulva with your mouth.
16. Take a few seconds to find your most comfortable position.

PAUSE A FEW SECONDS

17. Start by gently licking and nuzzling your partner's vulva and entire pubic area with your lips, tongue and nose.

PAUSE A FEW SECONDS

Notice your thoughts, self-talk, mental images and emotions about licking, sucking, and nuzzling your partner's vulva.

If your mind wanders into the future or the past or fills with unhelpful thoughts and feelings, note that this is happening and say to yourself, *there goes my runaway mind again, taking me out of the present moment,* and focus on your partner's vulva.

18. Notice the effects of your movements on your partner's vulva and the rest of her body.

PAUSE A FEW SECONDS

19. Now part your partner's vaginal lips with your fingers and gently stimulate your partner's vaginal lips with your tongue.

PAUSE A FEW SECONDS

20. Use your tongue to gently lick, flick, or swirl around your partner's vaginal lips, from her clitoris, to her perineum (the area between her vaginal opening and anal opening).

PAUSE A FEW SECONDS

21. After a few moments of doing this, change actions and insert your tongue into your partner's vagina.
22. Explore your partner's vaginal opening by pushing your tongue into the opening and swirling it around.

PAUSE A FEW SECONDS

23. Take your time and notice your partner's vulva and vaginal opening as you lick, swirl, and probe it with your tongue.

PAUSE A FEW SECONDS

24. After a few moments of doing this change actions and gently suck on your partner's vaginal lips. Use your tongue and lips to suck on your partner's entire vaginal lips.

Notice your thoughts, self-talk, mental images and emotions as you lick and suck your partner's vaginal lips and insert your tongue into her vagina.

If your mind wanders into the future or the past or fills with unhelpful thoughts and feelings, note that this is happening and say to yourself, *there goes my runaway mind again, taking me out of the present moment*, and focus on your partner's vulva.

25. Part her vaginal lips and gently find her clitoris. Notice the size, shape, texture, and taste of her clitoris as you gently lick and suck it.

PAUSE A FEW SECONDS

26. The clitoris contains the most nerve endings of her entire vulva, so spend time licking, sucking, and caressing this area with your lips, tongue, nose and face.

PAUSE A FEW SECONDS

27. Notice the effects of your licking, sucking, and nuzzling on your partner.
28. Notice any changes to the size, shape, and color of your partner's vulva in this aroused state.

PAUSE A FEW SECONDS

29. Now back off and massage your partner's vulva with your hand for a while. Use your entire hand to cup her vulva in your hand and massage it with a circular motion, keeping firm but gentle pressure on her clitoris.
30. As you do this, relax, and enjoy what you are doing rather than thinking about what you "should" be doing. Notice the effects of your actions on your partner.

PAUSE A FEW SECONDS

31. Take this opportunity to ask your partner if you are applying the right amount of pressure with your mouth and face when you lick, suck, and nuzzle her vulva.
32. Ask her if she wants you to continue to insert one or more fingers into her vagina as you lick and suck on her clitoris and vaginal lips.
33. If she wants it, insert one or more fingers and gently thrust them in and out as you lick and suck on her vulva.

PAUSE A FEW SECONDS

34. Continue to lick, suck, and nuzzle your partner's clitoris, vaginal lips, and vaginal opening, adjusting the pressure, intensity, and speed of your actions based on what your partner told you she desires.

PAUSE A FEW SECONDS

35. If you are comfortable with it, lick your partner's perineum, the area between your partner's vaginal opening and her anal opening. This area is an often overlooked erogenous zone.

36. Spend a few moments licking this area.

PAUSE A FEW SECONDS

Notice your thoughts, self-talk, mental images and emotions as you lick and suck your partner's vaginal lips and her perineum.

If your mind wanders into the future or the past or fills with unhelpful thoughts and feelings, note that this is happening and say to yourself, *there goes my runaway mind again, taking me out of the present moment*, and focus on your partner's vulva.

37. At this point, your partner might start moving her vulva against your face as she might be getting ready to come.
38. Notice what is going on in her vulva, legs, and the rest of her body as she gets ready to orgasm.
39. Her legs will start tensing, her toes will start curling, and other muscles will get tighter and more tense. Her breathing will also increase. She might start to arch her back and push even more forcefully against your lips, tongue, and face.

PAUSE A FEW SECONDS

40. If your partner is ready to come, you can finish her off with your lips, tongue, face and fingers.
41. If she isn't ready, relax, and continue with whatever motions you wish until your partner comes.

PAUSE A FEW SECONDS

Notice your thoughts, self-talk, mental images and emotions as you bring your partner to orgasm.

If your mind wanders into the future or the past or fills with unhelpful thoughts and feelings note that this is happening and say to yourself, *there goes my runaway mind again, taking me out of the present moment*, and focus on your partner's vulva and her orgasm.

42. Spend a few moments maintaining contact with your partner as she finishes having her orgasm.

PAUSE A FEW SECONDS

43. When she is finished coming, relax, curl up with your partner and just cuddle for a while.

CHAPTER 17

Sexual Intercourse as a Gourmet Meal

The term sexual intercourse implies that two different types of connections occur when you have sex with your partner: (1) there is a sexual connection and (2) there is an interpersonal one. This is what makes sexual intercourse different from—and not necessarily better than—masturbation, autoeroticism, and sexual fantasy. You cannot have sexual intercourse without some type of connection to your partner. Even the most casual form of sexual intercourse, the one night stand, makes it an encounter with another human being, and therefore it is a social experience as well as a sexual one.

While this may seem so obvious, it is important to appreciate the social aspect of sexual intercourse because it creates an entirely different set of thoughts, self-talk, mental images, and then sex with yourself. The addition of another human being and the social dimension of sexual intercourse creates an entirely new perspective for you to be mindful of. The following section is not intended to be an exhaustive review of sexual intercourse positions. It is intended to get you thinking about your thoughts, self-talk, mental images and emotions related to sexual intercourse. It is also designed to reveal the subtle differences a position can make, not only in terms of sexual pleasure, but in what your mind is telling you. Hopefully, this will help you to begin to form new, more helpful sexual thoughts, self-talk, mental images, and emotions about them.

Vaginal Intercourse

Vaginal intercourse is also known as coitus and is one of the most common forms of sexual activity. The three starting points for vaginal intercourse are face-to-face, side-by-side, and rear entry. Using the term, "starting point" rather than "position" will help you understand that each starting point offers a limitless array of positions depending on how you place the rest of your body (arms, legs, torso, and so on).

Face-to-face positions have two variations: woman on top and man on top. If you are a woman, the woman-on-top position allows you greater control in the depth, pace, and motion of your partner's thrusting. It gives you the greatest control in clitoral stimulation and is the easiest intercourse position for you to manually stimulate your clitoris if you wish to. Orgasm rates for heterosexual women using the woman-on-top position are better than for any other position. This position is also good for helping heterosexual male partners control premature ejaculation.

The man-on-top position is also known as the "missionary position." If you are a man with sexual intercourse experience, you are probably used to this position as it is the most commonly used intercourse position in the United States. In this position you lie on top of your partner and you or your partner spreads her vaginal lips and inserts your penis into her vagina. You support your weight on your elbows, hands, knees, or across your partner's entire body as your penis moves in her vagina.

The most typical penile movements involve thrusting in and out as your partner either remains still or moves her hips in concert with her partner's thrusting. These motions provide direct sexual stimulation of the nerve endings on the shaft, glans, and corona (head) of your penis. Your partner's clitoris usually is stimulated as her clitoral hood, the top of her vaginal lips (the labia minora), pulls back and forth over it or your pubic area rubs against it. The vagina is stimulated as the penis slides in and out. The deeper recesses of the vagina (cervical area) may or may not be stimulated depending on the depth of the strokes and the positions. An option to thrusting in and out is a circular motion, known as grinding, which involves more pubis-to-pubis contact and stimulates your partner's clitoris differently. This provides more direct and intense stimulation of the clitoris and the base of your penis and can be done even after you have ejaculated (as long as you stop thrusting, which will dislodge your penis).

Variations of this starting point involve changing the position of the legs and arms. Your partner can experience a variety of different sensations and depths of penetration by wrapping her legs around your ankles, legs, or waist. Or she can throw her legs over your shoulders as you thrust in and out, which affords the deepest penetration. One of the advantages of this position is that it allows you to look into your partner's eyes and communicate. It also allows you and your partner to rub and caress each other's torsos and genitals. Furthermore, it allows use of the hands to enhance stimulation by touching or rubbing the partner's genitals during intercourse.

The rear entry starting point is also known as "doggie style" because it is the way in which dogs and most other animals have intercourse. If you are a man, in the rear entry position you would enter your partner's vagina from behind. If you are a woman this is usually accomplished by you kneeling on your hands and knees and your partner kneeling behind you, either between or straddling your legs. Either you or your partner can part your vaginal lips and guides the penis in.

This position creates deep vaginal penetration but little direct clitoral stimulation. For this reason, either you or your partner can stimulate your clitoris manually. This position also offers stimulation of the anus and perineum (the skin between the anal and vaginal openings) through pressure and friction from your partner's pubis rubbing or grinding against it. Two other rear entry position variations are (1) you can lie down with the man on top of the woman, or (2) you can lie on your sides. The latter is commonly known as the "spoon" position. One disadvantage of this position is that the partners do not face each other, which makes communication and kissing more difficult.

The side-to-side vaginal intercourse can involve face-to-face positioning or rear entry positioning. Because neither you nor your partner are bearing the full weight of the other, the side-to-side position is ideal for leisurely lovemaking or the rest period between more vigorous sessions. The easiest way to get into the side-to-side position is by rolling into it from the man-on-top or woman-on-top or the rear entry position.

Anal Intercourse

Straight and gay couples both practice anal intercourse. If you are a heterosexual man, you insert your penis into your partner's anus and rectum. If you are a homosexual man you may be the insertive or receptive partner. Like vaginal intercourse, anal intercourse can take place from the three starting points: side-to-side, rear entry, or face-to-face. The advantages and disadvantages associated with these starting points for vaginal intercourse are similar to those for anal intercourse. Rear entry is the most commonly used starting point for anal intercourse, although anal penetration can be accomplished through all of the positions previously described

Mindful Sexual Intercourse Exercise #1: Sex As a Gourmet Meal

Purpose: For many people, sex is a race with both partners competing to see who crosses the finish line with an orgasm. Even better, both partners cross at the same time and have the ultimate prize—mutual orgasms. Instead of a competition, I think of sex as more of a multicourse gourmet meal. With each course the couple anticipates something special, a unique taste delight. The purpose of this activity is to get couples to slow down and savor the process of lovemaking as much as the outcome.

The following is a set of preliminary instructions to use for all of the mindful sex activities.

1. Read the full instructions for whatever mindful sex activity you choose to engage in before doing it with your partner.
2. This will ensure that there are no surprises and you are comfortable with the instructions.
3. Allow 30 minutes of uninterrupted time for each activity.
4. Do this and all of the other mindful sex activities in the bedroom on your own bed.
5. Make sure the room is at a temperature that you and your partner find relaxing.
6. Put relaxing background music on that will help cancel out distracting sounds from the outside environment.
7. Make sure that the music you choose is instrumental and has no singing. Songs tend to distract your mind and take the focus off of the activity and onto thinking about the music.
8. Turn off your cell phone, television, and any distracting device.
9. Burn your favorite scented candle or incense.
10. Take a shower or bath with your partner before engaging in any of these activities.
11. Be mindful of the warmth of the water, the smell and feel of your partner and the soap as you move it over your partner's body and get clean and ready for these mindful sex activities.
12. When performing this activity keep your mind on your partner's body. Focus your attention on what each motion feels like and how your partner responds to your actions.
13. When your mind drifts to the past or future, or starts "thinking" or "worrying" about if you are doings things right or perfect, just get back to noticing, without judgment, what each motion feels like and how your partner responds to your actions.

14. Whenever your mind drifts, say to yourself, *there goes my runaway mind again, taking me out of the present moment*, and shift your focus back on what you are doing to your partner.

That's it for general instructions. I will talk you through each activity, step by step. Relax and enjoy the process.

Specific Instructions:

1. Make sure you read and complete the preliminary instructions before proceeding.
2. Set aside one full hour of uninterrupted time for this activity.
3. Think of this one-hour lovemaking session as a gourmet meal.
4. Take your time with each course; savor it and do not rush.
5. Don't look at having an orgasm as the objective.
6. Don't even think beyond the course you are involved in, your actions, and those of your partner.
7. For course number one just relax in bed eating and drinking.

    - Don't get drunk or eat too much.
    - The idea is to have a sensual snack.
    - Think of the Mindful Eating and Drinking in Bed Activity you did and use this as a prelude to your lovemaking.

8. Give your partner a massage for a few minutes.

    - Have your partner choose which type of massage.
    - Take your time, use oil or powder, and be mindful of what is going on in your hands and body, your partner's body, and the bedroom environment.
    - Continue this for as long as you wish and then switch and have your partner massage you.

PAUSE FOR A FEW MOMENTS

As you continue to enjoy your massage, notice your thoughts, self-talk, mental images and feelings that accompany your massage.

When your mind wanders into the future or the past or fills up with unhelpful thoughts and feelings, note that this is happening and say to yourself, *there goes my runaway mind again, taking me out of the present moment*, and get back to the present moment.

9. After you have both massaged each other, pause and have a sip of wine and a piece of fruit.

10. Now shift your attention to your partner's vulva or penis and get into position to give your partner oral sex for a while.

    - Remember the basic movements for giving your partner oral sex; relax and take your time.
    - Pay attention to the sights, sounds, tastes, touch, and smell of giving your partner oral sex.

11. Ask your partner if there is anything they would like you to do to enhance the experience for them.

PAUSE A FEW SECONDS

As you continue to give your partner oral sex, notice your thoughts, self-talk, mental images and feelings that accompany giving your partner oral sex.

When your mind wanders into the future or the past or fills up with unhelpful thoughts and feelings, note that this is happening and say to yourself, *there goes my runaway mind again, taking me out of the present moment*, and get back to giving your partner oral sex.

12. Now switch and let your partner give you oral sex for a while.

    - Pay attention to the sights, sounds, tastes, touch, and smell of your partner giving you oral sex.

13. Tell your partner if there is anything you would like them to do to enhance the experience for you.

PAUSE A FEW SECONDS

As you continue to receive oral sex, notice your thoughts, self-talk, mental images, and feelings that accompany your partner going down on you.

When your mind wanders into the future or the past or fills up with unhelpful thoughts and feelings, note that this is happening and say to yourself, *there goes my runaway mind again, taking me out of the present moment*, and get back to focusing on your partner giving you oral sex."

14. If you both desire it, get into position and give each other oral sex for a while.

    - Pay attention to the sights, sounds, tastes, touch, and smell of giving and receiving oral sex.

15. Tell your partner if there is anything you would like them to do to enhance the experience for you.

PAUSE A FEW SECONDS

As you continue to give and receive oral sex, notice your thoughts, self-talk, mental images, and feelings that accompany this activity.

When your mind wanders into the future or the past or fills up with unhelpful thoughts and feelings, note that this is happening and say to yourself, *there goes my runaway mind again, taking me out of the present moment*, and get back to focusing on giving and receiving oral sex.

16. After a while, take a break and grab a sip of wine and a piece of fruit.
17. Feed your partner for a while and express your appreciation for such a wonderful love-making session.
18. Now shift your focus to sexual intercourse and ask your partner how they want to be entered or enter you.
19. After a while, change intercourse positions. I recommend finishing with one that your partner is most likely to achieve orgasm with.
20. Continue in this position until your partner comes.

PAUSE A FEW SECONDS

21. If you haven't come and want to, tell your partner what you will need in order to come.
22. Remember, you can have great sex even if you don't have an orgasm, so this is your choice.

PAUSE A FEW SECONDS

23. After you either have an orgasm or decide to stop having intercourse, don't pull out or have your partner pull out immediately.
24. Instead, just lie together, still connected, and enjoy the sensations involved in winding down and achieving resolution.

PAUSE A FEW SECONDS

As you continue to lie in your partner's arms notice your thoughts, self-talk, mental images, and feelings that accompany this activity.

Relax. You have nowhere to go, and nothing to do.

25. If you or your partner is using a condom, make sure to hold it firmly at the base of the penis when withdrawing it if it has gone limp. This will ensure that the condom doesn't spill the ejaculate into the vagina.

Epilogue

Well, that's it, you now have all the tools you need to start practicing sexual mindfulness with your partner. Remember, all of the formal (meditation etc.) and informal (Eight Shades Of ...etc.) techniques for building internal and external mindfulness are transformative. That is, if you practice them on a regular basis they will transform the way you live your life. Eventually they will influence the way you see yourself and the world around you. You start to notice, without judgment, the world around you.

Remember, becoming more mindful means relearning what you were born with: the ability to look at each day and each sexual experience with your partner with a beginner's mind. It is already in you. Take your time and enjoy the process of becoming more mindful as much as the outcome.

Good luck,

Dr Rich

PS: You might find my audio collection, *Sexual Mindfulness,* helpful. It has audio recordings of all of the sexual mindfulness exercises from chapters 14-17. You can listen to the step-by-step instructions to please your partner. Get yours from my website by going to:
https://www.drrichblonna.com/audio/sexual-mindfulness/

Reference List

Anderson, L. and Krech, G. (1996). *A finger pointing at the moon.* Monkton, VT: ToDo Institute.

Basson, R. (2000). The female sexual response: A different model. *Journal of Marital Therapy, 26,* 51–65.

Blonna, R., Carter, L. (2018). *Healthy Sexuality: 2nd Edition*. Dubuque IA: Hendall Hunt Publishing.

Blonna R, LoSchiavo, J, Watter, D. (2011). Health Counseling; A Microskills Approach for Counselors, Educators, and Nurses. Sudbury MA. Jones and Bartlett Publishers.

Blonna R, (2012). Coping With Stress in a Changing World, 5th Ed. NYC NY: McGraw-Hill Publishing.

Blonna, R. (2010). *Stress less, live more: How Acceptance and Commitment Therapy can help you live a busy yet balanced life.* Oakland, CA: New Harbinger Publications. Germer, C. (2005). Mindfulness: What is it? Does it matter? In Germer, C., Siegel, R., and Fulton, P. (Eds.). *Mindfulness and psychotherapy.* New York: Guilford Press.

Giles, GG, Severin, DR, English, MC, Credie, MR, Borland, R, Boyle, P. Hopper JL (2003). Sexual Factors and Prostate Cancer. BJU International 92, pp 211-216.

Harris, R. (2007). *The happiness trap.* Boston, MA: Trumpeter Press.

Hayes, S. (1984). Making sense of spirituality. *Behaviorism, 12:99-110.*

Hayes, S. (2005). *Get out of your mind and into your life.* Oakland, CA: New Harbinger Publications.

Hayes, S.C., Strosahl, K., and Wilson, K.G. (1999). *Acceptance and Commitment Therapy: An experiential approach to behavior change.* New York: Guilford Press.

Ivey AE, Gluckstern NB, Ivey MB (1997a). Basic Attending Skills 3rd. Edition(book). North Amherst Mass: Microtraining Associates.

Ivey AE, Gluckstern NB, Ivey MB (1997b). Basic Influencing Skills 3rd. Edition(videotape). North Amherst Mass: Microtraining Associates.

Kabat-Zinn, J (2013). Full Catastrophe Living: Using the Wisdom of Your Body and Mind to Face Stress, Pain, and Illness. New York: Bantam Books.

Kaplan, H. S. (1985). *Comprehensive evaluation of disorders of sexual desire.* Washington, DC: American Psychiatric Press.

Krech, G. (2005). *Working with your attention: Exercises and daily journal.* Monkton, VT: ToDo Institute.

Krech, G. (2002). *Naikan: Grace, gratitude, and the Japanese art of* Morita, S.

Laumann, EO, Gagnon, JH, Michael, RT, Michaels, S. (1994). The social organization of human sexuality: Sexual Practices in the United States. Chicago: University of Chicago Pres.

Morita, S (1998). Morita Therapy and the True Nature of Anxiety Disorders. Albany: State University of NY Press.

Nathan, J. (1990). Sitting, laboring, and changing: A critical examination of the indigenous Japanese psychotherapies. *Psychologia: An International Journal of Psychology in the Orient* , 33(3), pp. 163–170.

Masters, W., and Johnson, V. (1966). *Human sexual response.* Boston: Little, Brown.

Stayton, W. R. (2002, April–May). A theology of sexual pleasure. *SIECUS Report, 30*(4), 27–30.

Walen, S. R., and Roth, D. (1987). A cognitive approach to sex therapy. In J. H. Geer and W. T. O'Donohue (Eds.), *Theories of Human Sexuality.* New York: Plenum.

Yoshimoto, I. (1973). *A guide to Naikan.* Nara, Japan: Naikan Training Center Publications.

Manufactured by Amazon.ca
Bolton, ON

17994573R00148